Cardiac Arrhythmias

Cardiac Arrhythmias

Practical notes on interpretation and treatment

Sixth edition

David H. Bennett MD, FRCP, FACC, FESC
Consultant Cardiologist,
Regional Cardiac Centre,
Wythenshawe Hospital,
Manchester,
England

A member of the Hodder Headline Group
LONDON • NEW YORK • NEW DELHI

First published in Great Britain in 2002 by
Arnold, a member of the Hodder Headline Group,
338 Euston Road, London NW1 3BH

http://www.arnoldpublishers.com

Distributed in the United States of America by
Oxford University Press Inc.,
198 Madison Avenue, New York, NY10016
Oxford is a registered trademark of Oxford University Press

British Library Cataloguing in Publication Data
A catalogue record for this book is available from the British Library

Library of Congress Cataloging-in-Publication Data
A catalog record for this book is available from the Library of Congress

ISBN 0 340 80731 8

1 2 3 4 5 6 7 8 9 10

Publisher: Joanna Koster
Production Editor: James Rabson
Production Controller: Iain McWilliams
Cover Designer: Mouse Mat Design

Typeset in 9½ on 12 pt Palatino by Phoenix Photosetting, Chatham, Kent
Printed and bound in Malta by Gutenberg Press Ltd

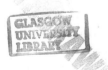

CONTENTS

The purpose of this sixth edition remains the same as its predecessors: to provide a practical guide to the diagnosis, investigation and management of the main cardiac arrhythmias with particular emphasis on the problems commonly faced in practice.

There have been important developments in the understanding and in the treatment of arrhythmias since the last edition. In particular, the applications of radiofrequency catheter ablation, pacemakers and implantable defibrillators have expanded, while the indications for antiarrhythmic drugs have diminished. Accordingly, the text has been updated and slightly expanded. There are many new electrocardiograms.

The quiz section has been revised and enlarged to provide a challenge to those who may be familiar with previous editions.

I would like to thank Dr Joanna Koster and her colleagues at Arnold for their help and expertise.

D.H.B.

PREFACE TO THE FIRST EDITION

The purpose of this book is to describe the main cardiac arrhythmias, with particular emphasis on the problems commonly encountered in their interpretation, and to discuss the practical aspects of current methods of investigation and treatment. Information of purely academic value has not been included. This book is intended to fill the gap between those textbooks that cover only the basics of arrhythmias and those that are written for the cardiac electrophysiologist. It has been written with junior hospital doctors in mind. They receive little formal training in the management of cardiac arrhythmias and yet, because prompt action is often required, the onus of diagnosis and treatment usually falls on them. It should also be of interest to medical students, who themselves will soon be responsible for dealing with arrhythmias, to nurses working in coronary and intensive care units and to physicians who want a brief review of the practical aspects of cardiac arrhythmias. I would like to thank the cardiac technicians, coronary care nurses and medical staff at Wythenshawe Hospital for their help. I am particularly grateful to my colleagues, Dr Colin Bray and Dr Christopher Ward. Thanks are also due to Mrs Mary Rooney for typing the manuscript and to the Wythenshawe Hospital Medical Illustration Department. Finally, I would like to acknowledge the distractions provided by my family, Irene, Samantha and Sally, to whom this book is dedicated.

The subject of cardiac arrhythmias may appear complex; and indeed some enjoy making it look complicated! However, there are only a dozen important disturbances of cardiac rhythm. They all have characteristic electrocardiographic appearances that in most cases are easily identifiable. So do not lose heart!

Remember, when assessing a cardiac rhythm, that only atrial and ventricular activity register on the surface electrocardiogram (ECG). The site of impulse formation, sequence of cardiac chamber activation and functions of the sinus node and atrioventricular junction have to be deduced from analysis of the atrial and ventricular electrograms.

A single 'rhythm strip' may be inadequate for diagnosis. Scrutiny of several ECG leads, preferably recorded simultaneously, may be necessary. For example, atrial activity is often the key to diagnosis but may not be clearly shown in all ECG leads: it is often best seen in leads II and V1. Often, a '12-lead ECG' will provide much more information than a rhythm strip.

The electrocardiograms in this book have been recorded at the conventional paper speed of 25 mm/s, unless otherwise indicated. At this speed, each large square represents 0.2 s and each small square represents 0.04 s. Heart rate (beats/min) can therefore be calculated by dividing the number of large squares between two consecutive complexes into 300, or by dividing the number of small squares between two complexes into 1500.

An ECG recorded during an arrhythmia that is of diagnostic importance should always be safely stored in the patient's notes. This guideline, which may be very important to the long-term management of a patient, is often ignored, particularly on intensive care units!

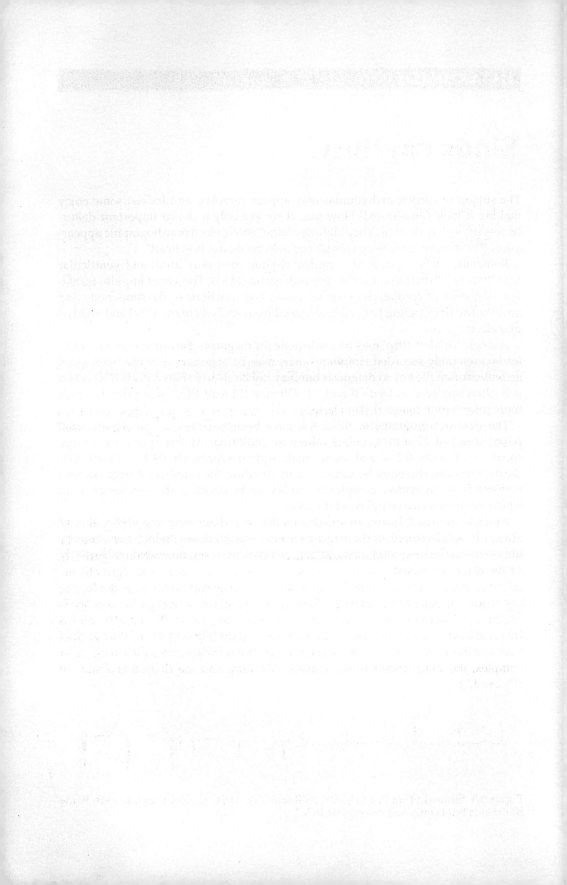

Sinus rhythm

ECG CHARACTERISTICS

The sinus node initiates the electrical impulse that activates atrial and then ventricular myocardium during each normal heartbeat. Sinus node activity itself does not register on the electrocardiogram (ECG).

P WAVE

Atrial activity, the P wave, is usually apparent in most ECG leads (Figure 1.1). However, sometimes the P wave is not visible or is of low amplitude, and it may be necessary to inspect all leads of the ECG to establish there is sinus rhythm (Figure 1.2).

The sinus node lies at the junction of the superior vena cava and right atrium. Atrial activation spreads from the sinus node inferiorly (that is towards the feet) to the atrioventricular (AV) junction. The P wave, therefore, is upright in those leads which are directed to the inferior surface of the heart, i.e. II, III and aVF, and is inverted in aVR, which faces the superior heart surface (Figure 1.1). If a P wave does not have these characteristics then, even though a P wave precedes each ventricular complex, the sinus node has not activated the atria and the rhythm is abnormal (Figure 1.3).

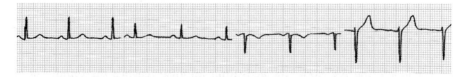

Figure 1.1 Sinus rhythm (leads I, aVF, aVR and V2). Atrial activity is clearly seen in the limb leads but is only just discernible in V2

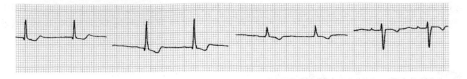

Figure 1.2 Sinus rhythm with low-amplitude P waves (leads I, II, III and V1). Atrial activity is only clearly seen in V1

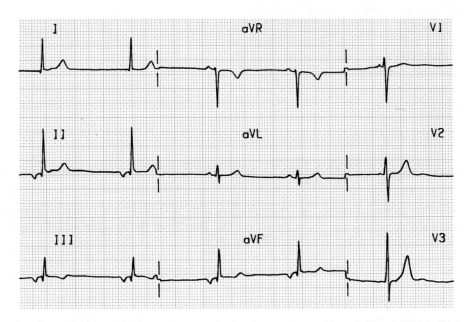

Figure 1.3 Junctional rhythm: a P wave precedes each QRS complex but is superiorly directed. It is negative in leads II, III and aVF

PR INTERVAL

The AV node delays conduction of the atrial impulse to the ventricles. Conduction through the AV node does not register on the ECG. The PR interval, which is measured from the onset of the P wave to the onset of the ventricular complex, indicates the time taken for an atrial impulse to reach the ventricles. The normal PR interval ranges from 0.12 to 0.21 s. It should shorten during sinus tachycardia.

QRS COMPLEX

After traversing the AV node, the activating impulse reaches the bundle of His which divides into the right and left bundle branches. The bundle of His, the bundle branches and their ramifications, the Purkinje fibres, constitute the 'specialized intraventricular conducting system' which facilitates very rapid conduction of the impulse through the ventricular myocardium. Ventricular activation is represented by the QRS complex which is normally less than 0.08 s in duration.

Table 1.1 The characteristics of normal sinus rhythm

P wave:
    Precedes each QRS complex
    Upright in leads III, aVF
    Inverted in lead aVR

PR interval:
    Duration 0.12–0.21 s

QRS complex:
    Duration less than 0.08 s

SINUS BRADYCARDIA

Sinus bradycardia is sinus rhythm at a rate less than 60 beats/min (Figure 1.4). It may be physiological, as in athletes or during sleep, or may result from acute myocardial infarction, sick sinus syndrome or from drugs such as beta-adrenoceptor blocking drugs. Non-cardiac disorders such as myxoedema, jaundice and raised intracranial pressure can also cause sinus bradycardia.

Atropine or pacing can be used to increase the rate but are only necessary when sinus bradycardia causes symptoms, marked hypotension or leads to tachy-arrhythmia.

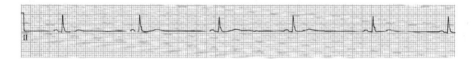

Figure 1.4 Sinus bradycardia (lead II): rate 34 beats/min

SINUS TACHYCARDIA

This is defined as sinus rhythm at a rate greater than 100 beats/min (Figure 1.5). Exercise, anxiety or any disorder that increases sympathetic nervous system activity may cause sinus tachycardia. Occasionally it may be due to a primary disorder of the sinus node (sinus node re-entry).

Since sinus tachycardia is usually a physiological response, there is rarely a need for specific treatment. However, if sinus tachycardia is inappropriate, the rate may be slowed by beta-adrenoceptor blocking drugs.

At rest, the sinus node rate is seldom above 100 beats/min unless the patient is very ill. In contrast, atrial flutter with 2:1 AV block often leads to a heart rate of 140–160 beats/min and can easily be mistaken for sinus tachycardia (*see* chapter 7).

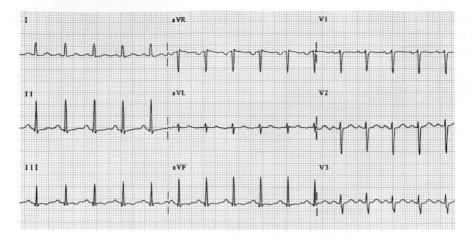

Figure 1.5 Sinus tachycardia during exercise: rate 136 beats/min

SINUS ARRHYTHMIA

Normally there are only minor changes in rate during sinus rhythm. In sinus arrhythmia, which is of no pathological significance, there are alternating periods of slowing and increasing sinus node rate. Usually the rate increases during inspiration (Figure 1.6). Sinus arrhythmia is most commonly seen in the young.

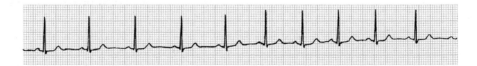

Figure 1.6 Sinus arrhythmia

Main points

- During sinus rhythm, an inferiorly directed P wave (i.e. upright in leads III and aVF) precedes each QRS complex.

- If AV conduction is normal, the duration of the PR interval will be between 0.12 and 0.21 s.

- Normal intraventricular conduction results in a QRS complex with a duration less than 0.08 s.

- In cases of apparent sinus tachycardia at rest, exclude atrial flutter or tachycardia.

CHAPTER 2

Ectopic beats

PREMATURITY

The terms ectopic beat, extrasystole and premature contraction are, for practical purposes, synonymous. They refer to an impulse originating from the atria, AV junction (i.e. AV node plus bundle of His) or ventricles, which arises prematurely in the cardiac cycle (Figures 2.1–2.3).

By definition, an ectopic beat must arise earlier in the cardiac cycle than the next normally timed beat would be expected. Thus the interval between the ectopic beat and the preceding beat (i.e. the coupling interval) is shorter than the cycle length of the dominant rhythm. If this fact is ignored, other beats with abnormal

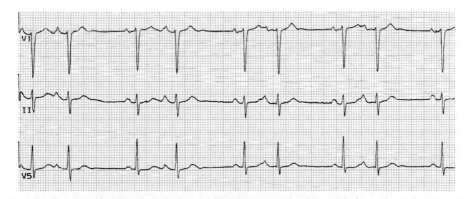

Figure 2.1 The second, fourth, sixth and eighth complexes are atrial ectopic beats. The ectopic P waves are premature and differ slightly in shape from those of sinus origin

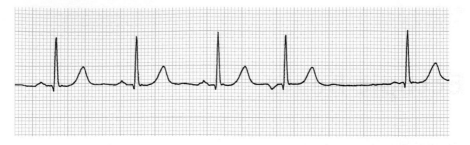

Figure 2.2 The fourth beat is a junctional ectopic beat (lead III). The junctional focus has activated the atria as well as the ventricles, resulting in an inverted P wave which precedes the QRS complex

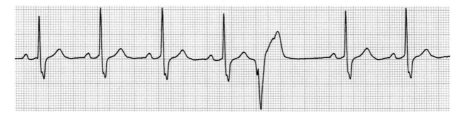

Figure 2.3 The fifth beat is a ventricular ectopic beat

configurations such as escape beats (*see* Chapter 3) and intermittent bundle branch block may be misinterpreted as ectopic beats.

The site of origin of an ectopic beat can be determined by careful examination of the ECG. A single rhythm strip may be inadequate. Scrutiny of simultaneous recordings of several ECG leads is often necessary to detect the diagnostic clues (Figures 2.4 and 2.5).

ATRIAL ECTOPIC BEATS

P WAVE

An atrial ectopic beat results in a P wave which is premature. The site of origin and therefore direction of atrial activation will differ from that during sinus rhythm so a premature P wave will usually differ in shape to a P wave of sinus node origin (Figure 2.1).

Because atrial ectopic beats are premature, they may be superimposed on and thus deform the T wave of the preceding beat. Careful examination of the ECG is essential to detect ectopic P waves; often, lead V1 is the best lead (Figures 2.5 and 2.6).

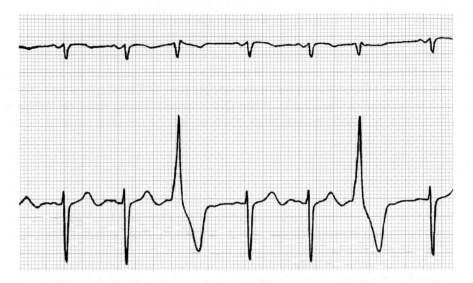

Figure 2.4 Simultaneous recording of leads V1 and V2. The third and sixth beats are unifocal ventricular ectopic beats. Their ventricular origin is not apparent in lead V1 but is obvious in V2

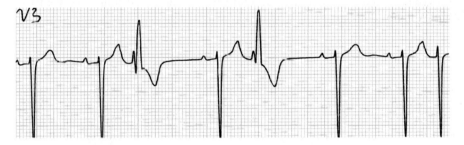

Figure 2.5 Atrial ectopic beats are superimposed on the T waves of the second, fourth and seventh ventricular complexes (lead V3). It can be seen how the T waves of these beats are modified by comparing them with the T wave of the first and sixth ventricular complexes which are not followed by an atrial ectopic. The first two atrial ectopic beats are conducted with right bundle branch block

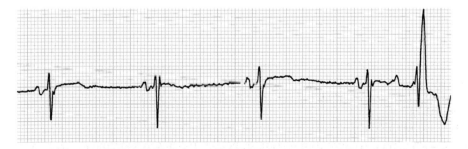

Figure 2.6 The last beat is an atrial ectopic beat conducted with first-degree AV block and right bundle branch block.

AV AND INTRAVENTRICULAR CONDUCTION

Usually the AV junction and bundle branches will conduct an atrial ectopic beat to the ventricles in the same manner as if the sinus node had activated the atria. Thus the PR interval and QRS complex of the ectopic beat will be identical with those during sinus rhythm (Figure 2.1). If the QRS complex during sinus rhythm was abnormal due to bundle branch block, then so will be the QRS complex of the ectopic beat.

Sometimes, however, atrial ectopic beats, especially those that arise very early in the cardiac cycle, may encounter either an AV junction or a bundle branch which has not yet recovered from conduction of the last atrial impulse and is, therefore, partially or completely refractory to excitation. Partial and complete refractoriness of the AV junction will result in prolongation of the PR interval and blocked atrial ectopic beats, respectively (Figures 2.6–2.8). Blocked atrial ectopics have been wrongly taken as an indication for cardiac pacing!

Partial or complete refractoriness of one or other bundle branch (it is usually the right bundle) will correspondingly lead to partial or complete bundle branch block (Figures 2.6 and 2.7). This phenomenon of functional bundle branch block is referred to by some as 'phasic aberrant intraventricular conduction'. The resultant QRS complexes are broad and can therefore be confused with ventricular ectopic beats if the premature P wave preceding the ventricular complex is not detected.

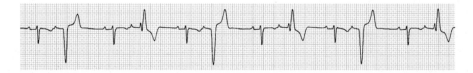

Figure 2.7 Lead V1. Atrial ectopic beats follow each sinus beat. The second, sixth and tenth complexes are atrial ectopic beats conducted with left bundle branch block. The fourth, eighth and twelfth complexes are conducted with right bundle branch block.

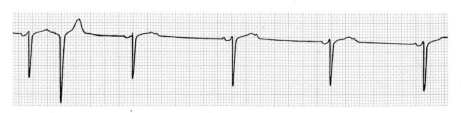

Figure 2.8 Lead V1. Atrial ectopic beats are superimposed on the terminal portion of the T wave of each ventricular complex. The first atrial ectopic is conducted with partial left branch block. The other atrial ectopic beats are not conducted to the ventricles

Table 2.1 Characteristics of atrial ectopic beats

The P wave:
  Will be premature
  May be superimposed on and distort the preceding T wave
  Will usually be followed by a normal QRS complex
  May sometimes not be conducted to the ventricles, or be
  conducted with a bundle branch block pattern

SIGNIFICANCE

Atrial ectopic beats occur in many cardiac disorders but are also commonly found in individuals with normal hearts, particularly the elderly. They are usually benign. However, if they are frequent they may herald atrial fibrillation or atrial tachycardia.

AV JUNCTIONAL ECTOPIC BEATS

AV junctional beats used to be called 'nodal' beats. It is now recognized that at least part of the AV node is not capable of pacemaker activity and that it is not possible to distinguish between beats of AV nodal and His bundle origin. Hence the more general term 'AV junction'. AV junctional ectopic beats are not as common as atrial or ventricular ectopics. Treatment is rarely necessary.

ECG APPEARANCE

AV junctional ectopic beats are recognized by a premature QRS complex which is similar in appearance to that occurring in sinus rhythm. The junctional focus may activate the atria as well as the ventricles, leading to a retrograde P wave (i.e. negative in leads II, III and AVF). The retrograde P wave may precede, follow or be buried within the QRS complex, depending on the relative speeds of conduction of the premature junctional impulse to the ventricles and to the atria (Figure 2.2).

VENTRICULAR ECTOPIC BEATS

The impulse of a ventricular ectopic beat is not conducted through the ventricles via the specialized, rapidly conducting tissues.

ECG APPEARANCE

These result in a premature ventricular complex which is broad (>0.12 s), bizarre in shape and, in contrast to atrial ectopic beats, will obviously *not* be preceded by an ectopic P wave (Figures 2.3 and 2.4). The bizarre shape and prolonged duration of the ventricular complex reflect the abnormal course and consequent slowing of ventricular activation.

Several terms used to describe the origin, timing and quantity of ventricular ectopic beats are explained below.

Table 2.2 Characteristics of ventricular ectopic beats

The QRS complex of ventricular ectopic beats:
Will be premature
Will be broad (> 0.12 s)
Will be abnormal in shape
Will not be preceded by a premature P wave

Focus

Ectopic beats with the same shape and coupling intervals are assumed to arise from the same focus and are termed unifocal (Figure 2.4), whereas differing shapes and coupling intervals suggest more than one focus, i.e. multifocal or multiform (Figure 2.9).

Timing

Beats that occur very early in the cardiac cycle will be superimposed on the T wave of the preceding beat and are described as 'R on T' (Figure 2.10). Most episodes of

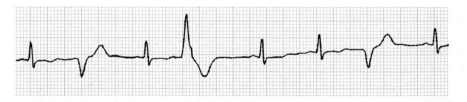

Figure 2.9 Multifocal ventricular ectopic beats. The second ventricular ectopic beat has a different shape and coupling interval from the first and third ectopic beats

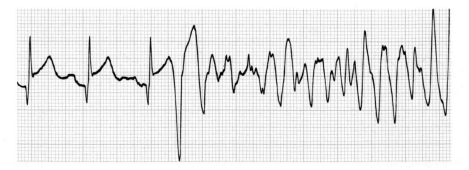

Figure 2.10 An 'R on T' ventricular ectopic beat which, in this case, initiates ventricular fibrillation

ventricular fibrillation and many episodes of ventricular tachycardia are initiated by 'R on T' ectopics; though by no means do all 'R on T' ectopic beats precipitate these arrhythmias.

A ventricular ectopic beat that occurs only slightly prematurely in the cardiac cycle may fall, by chance, immediately after a P wave initiated by normal sinus node activity: the P wave will therefore, in contrast to an atrial ectopic beat, not be premature. Such a ventricular ectopic beat is described as 'end-diastolic' (Figures 2.11 and 2.12).

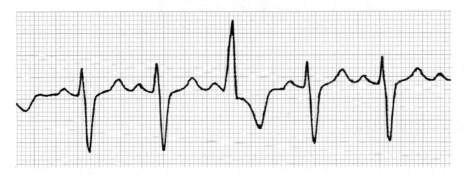

Figure 2.11 The third beat is an end-diastolic ventricular ectopic beat. It is preceded by a normally timed P wave

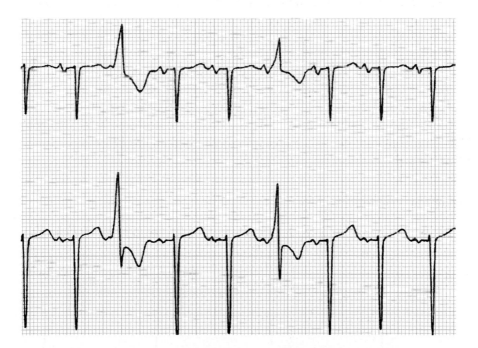

Figure 2.12 Simultaneous recording of leads V1 and V2. Two end-diastolic ventricular ectopic beats. The second mimicking the Wolff–Parkinson–White syndrome

Usually there is a pause after a ventricular ectopic beat. When there is no such pause and the ectopic beat is thus sandwiched between two normal beats, the ectopic beat is said to be 'interpolated' (Figure 2.13).

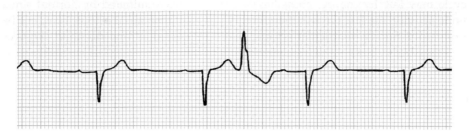

Figure 2.13 Interpolated ventricular beat. (The subsequent PR interval is prolonged owing to retrograde concealed conduction)

Quantification

Ventricular ectopic beats are often quantified by the number occurring each minute.

When an ectopic beat follows each sinus beat the term bigeminy is applied (Figure 2.14). If an ectopic follows a pair of normal beats there is trigeminy (Figure 2.15). When two ectopics occur in succession (Figure 2.16) they are referred to as a couplet. A salvo refers to more than two ectopic beats in succession.

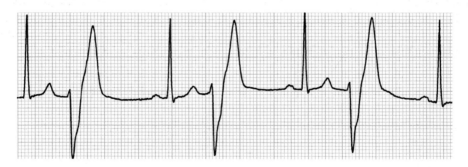

Figure 2.14 Ventricular bigeminy

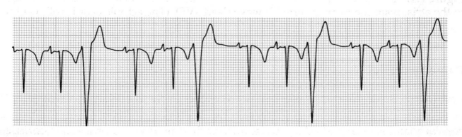

Figure 2.15 Ventricular trigeminy

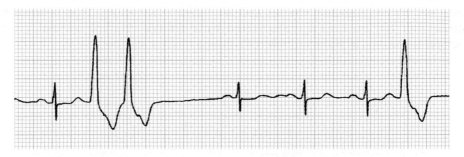

Figure 2.16 The first sinus beat is followed by a couplet of ventricular ectopic beats

Atrial activity

The pattern of atrial activity following a ventricular ectopic beat depends on whether the AV junction transmits the ventricular impulse to the atria. If this occurs, the result is an inverted P wave which is often superimposed on and may therefore be concealed by the ventricular ectopic beat (Figure 2.17). When the AV junction does not transmit the ventricular impulse to the atria, atrial activity continues independently of ventricular activity; it is only in these cases that a ventricular impulse is followed by a full compensatory pause, i.e. the lengths of the cycles before and after the ectopic beat will equal twice the sinus cycle length (see Figures 2.3 and 2.4).

Sometimes a ventricular impulse only partially penetrates the AV junction. The next impulse arising from the sinus node may therefore encounter an AV junction, which is partially refractory, and be conducted with a prolonged PR interval (Figure 2.13). This phenomenon of 'retrograde concealed conduction' often occurs following interpolated ventricular extrasystoles.

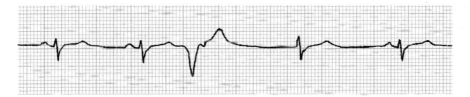

Figure 2.17 The third beat is a ventricular ectopic beat which has been conducted back to the atria, resulting in an inverted P wave (lead aVF). (The ectopic beat is followed by a junctional escape beat)

Parasystole

Parasystole, which is uncommon, is an exception to the rule that unifocal ectopic beats have a constant coupling interval. The ventricular ectopic focus discharges regularly and is undisturbed by the dominant rhythm. It will capture the ventricles provided the ectopic discharge does not occur when the ventricles have just been activated by the dominant rhythm and are therefore refractory. Thus ventricular parasystole (Figure 2.18) is characterized by a variable coupling interval, inter-ectopic intervals which are multiples of a common factor and, because the ventricles may by chance be simultaneously activated by both ectopic and normal pacemakers, fusion beats (i.e. a complex which is a composite of normal and ectopic beat).

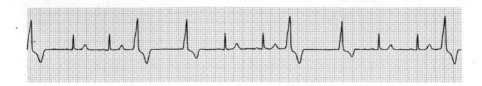

Figure 2.18 Ventricular parasystole. The ectopic beats have variable coupling intervals. The intervals between ectopic beats are multiples of 1.18 s. The fifth and ninth complexes are fusion beats

CAUSES AND SIGNIFICANCE OF VENTRICULAR ECTOPIC BEATS

Causes include acute myocardial infarction, myocardial ischaemia, myocardial damage caused by previous infarction, myocarditis or cardiomyopathy, mitral valve prolapse, valvular heart disease and digoxin toxicity.

Occasional ventricular ectopic beats at rest and even frequent unifocal ectopic beats on exercise occur in otherwise normal individuals and are not necessarily pathological or of prognostic significance. However, a recent large survey of middle-aged men did show that frequent ventricular ectopic beats (more than 10% of all ventricular complexes) occuring during exercise was associated with a 2.5 increase in mortality over the 23-year period of the survey. The frequency of ectopic beats in the adult population increases with age.

'Complex' ventricular ectopic beats – i.e. frequent, multifocal, 'R on T' or those that occur in salvos – are rarely found in the absence of cardiac disease and are associated with an increased cardiovascular mortality. In patients who have sustained myocardial damage from coronary heart disease, there is a correlation between severity of damage and frequency of ventricular ectopic beats. Recent evidence, however, points to the presence of ectopic beats as an added and independent risk factor, but there is no evidence to show that suppression of ectopic beats by anti-arrhythmic therapy improves prognosis. Indeed, several anti-arrhythmic drugs have been shown to increase mortality in patients with ventricular ectopic beats after myocardial infarction.

Usually, ectopic beats do not cause symptoms. Some patients, however, experience distressing symptoms. They may be upset by the irregularity resulting from the premature beats or by the compensatory pause or 'thump' caused by increased myocardial contractility associated with the post-ectopic beat. They may be anxious that their irregular heart rhythm is a sign of impending heart attack or other major cardiac problem.

There is a group of patients with structurally normal hearts who have distressing symptoms caused by ventricular ectopic beats in whom reassurance is inadequate.

In these patients, anti-arrhythmic therapy may be necessary for symptomatic purposes.

The significance of ventricular ectopic beats in acute myocardial infarction is discussed later.

Main points

- Ectopic beats are premature and therefore have a coupling interval shorter than the cycle length of the dominant rhythm.

- The P waves of atrial ectopic beats are often superimposed on and distort the preceding T wave and can easily be missed. They are usually best seen in lead VI.

- Atrial ectopic beats may sometimes not be conducted to the ventricles or may be conducted with a bundle branch block pattern.

- Ventricular ectopic beats cause premature, broad and bizarrely shaped QRS complexes. They are only followed by a full compensatory pause if they are not conducted to the atria.

- Chronic ventricular ectopic beats which are frequent, multifocal, 'R on T' or occur in salvos are associated with an increased cardiovascular mortality but there is no evidence to show that their suppression improves prognosis.

CHAPTER 3

Escape beats

TIMING

When the dominant pacemaker, usually the sinus node, fails to discharge, escape beats may arise from subsidiary sites in the specialized conducting system. In contrast to ectopic beats, escape beats are always late, i.e. the coupling interval is greater than the cycle length of the dominant rhythm (Figures 3.1 and 3.3). Distinction between escape and ectopic beats is important because the former indicate impaired pacemaker function. Escape beats themselves require no treatment. If treatment is necessary, it is to accelerate the basic rhythm.

ORIGINS

Escape beats usually arise from the AV junction (Figures 3.1–3.3); less commonly, they originate from the ventricles. The ventricular complexes of junctional escape

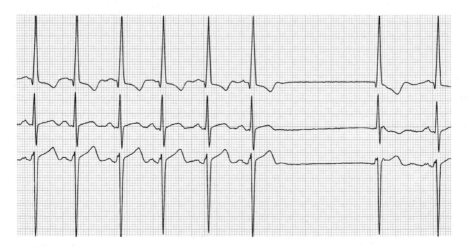

Figure 3.1 Leads I, II, III. After the sixth complex there is a pause in sinus node activity followed by a junctional escape beat

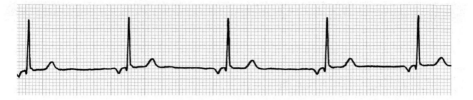

Figure 3.2 Junctional escape rhythm (lead II). The junctional focus has also activated the atria as indicated by the inverted P wave preceding each QRS complex

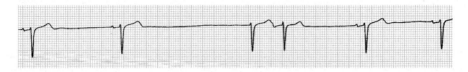

Figure 3.3 The third ventricular complex is a junctional escape beat which arises during sinus arrest. The escape beat is followed by an atrial ectopic beat

beats are similar to those during normal rhythm. As with junctional ectopic beats, the junctional focus may activate the atria as well as the ventricles, leading to a retrograde P wave (i.e. negative in leads II, III and aVF). The retrograde P wave may precede, follow or be buried within the QRS complex, depending on the relative speeds of conduction of the premature junctional impulse to the ventricles and to the atria.

Ventricular escape beats have a similar configuration to ventricular ectopic beats (Figures 3.4 and 3.5).

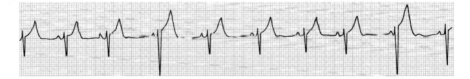

Figure 3.4 The fourth and ninth ventricular complexes are escape beats (probably arising from the ventricles) which result from slowing of the sinus node. Though P waves precede the escape beats, they are unlikely to have captured the ventricles since the PR intervals are shorter than those during sinus rhythm

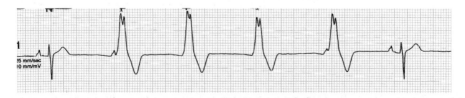

Figure 3.5 Ventricular escape rhythm during sinus bradycardia

Main points

- In contrast to ectopic beats, the coupling interval of escape beats is greater than the cycle length of the dominant rhythm.
- As with ectopic beats, the configuration of escape beats indicates whether they are of supraventricular or ventricular origin.
- Escape beats should not be suppressed by drugs.

CHAPTER 4

Bundle branch blocks

The bundle of His divides into left and right bundle branches. These facilitate the rapid activation of the left and right ventricles. The left bundle branch has two main subdivisions: the anterior and posterior fascicles.

RIGHT BUNDLE BRANCH BLOCK

ECG APPEARANCE

In right bundle branch block, there is delay in activation of the right ventricle while septal and left ventricular activation is normal (Figure 4.1). Delayed right ventricular activation results in:

1. an increase in duration of the QRS complex (> 0.12 s);
2. a secondary R wave in leads facing the right ventricle (V1 and V2) and hence an 'M'-shaped complex in these leads;
3. a broad S wave in left ventricular leads, especially lead I.

Partial right bundle branch block results in a similar ECG appearance but the QRS duration is 0.11 s or less.

CAUSES AND SIGNIFICANCE

Right bundle branch block may be an isolated congenital lesion. It often occurs in congenital heart disease, in other causes of right ventricular hypertrophy or strain

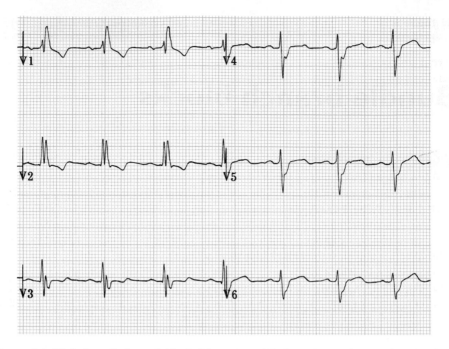

Figure 4.1 Right bundle branch block. There is an M-shaped complex in Vl and a deep slurred S wave in lead V6

and where there is myocardial damage. Right bundle branch block is common when there is disease of the specialized conducting tissues.

Supraventricular extrasystoles and tachycardias may encounter a right bundle branch which is refractory to excitation and be conducted to the ventricles with a right bundle branch block pattern.

Based on limited data, neither pre-existing nor acquired right bundle branch block are of prognostic significance.

LEFT BUNDLE BRANCH BLOCK

ECG APPEARANCE

In left bundle branch block, activation of the interventricular septum is in the opposite direction to normal being initiated by impulses arising from the right bundle branch. Thus:

1. the initial small negative Q wave normally seen in left ventricular leads (V5, V6, I and aVL) is replaced by a larger positive R wave.
2. activation of the left ventricle will be delayed, resulting in a secondary R wave in left ventricular leads and prolongation of the duration of the QRS complex (>0.12 s).

3. the primary and secondary R waves produce an M-shaped ventricular complex in left ventricular leads (Figure 4.2).

Partial left bundle branch block has a similar ECG appearance to complete left bundle branch block, but the QRS duration is 0.10 or 0.11 s.

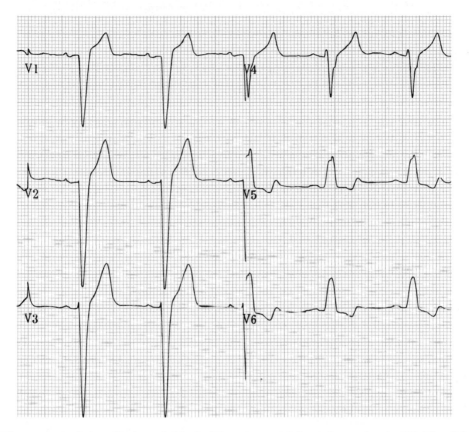

Figure 4.2 Left bundle branch block. There is an M-shaped complex in V6. The QS complex in V1 is also characteristic of left bundle branch block

CAUSES AND SIGNIFICANCE

Causes include myocardial damage due to coronary artery disease or cardio-myopathy, and left ventricular hypertrophy. Left bundle branch block can also be caused by disease of the specialized conduction tissues. Rarely, left bundle branch block may occur in an otherwise normal heart.

Supraventricular extrasystoles and tachycardias may encounter a left bundle branch which is refractory to excitation and be conducted to the ventricles with a left bundle branch block pattern.

Recently acquired left bundle branch block points to a poor prognosis.

Left bundle branch block can be intermittent (Figure 4.3).

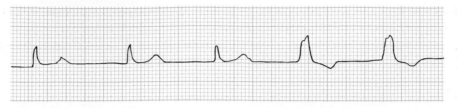

Figure 4.3 Intermittent left bundle branch block (lead aVL)

LEFT ANTERIOR AND POSTERIOR FASCICULAR BLOCKS

The anterior and posterior fascicles of the left bundle branch conduct impulses to the anterosuperior and posteroinferior regions of the left ventricle, respectively. Block can occur in either anterior or posterior fascicles and is known as fascicular block or hemiblock. Left anterior and posterior fascicular blocks are common in conduction tissue disease (*see* chapter 15).

Diagnosis of the fascicular blocks is based on the hexaxial reference system.

HEXAXIAL REFERENCE SYSTEM

The hexaxial reference system is a method of displaying the orientation of the six ECG limb leads to the heart in the frontal plane (Figure 4.4). For example, a superiorly directed impulse will move away from leads II, III and aVF, producing a negative wave in these leads, and towards aVL, producing a positive wave in this

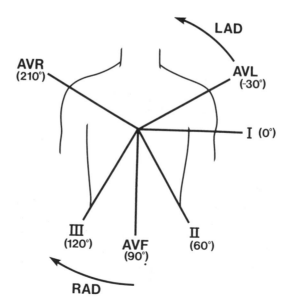

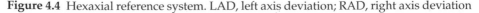

Figure 4.4 Hexaxial reference system. LAD, left axis deviation; RAD, right axis deviation

lead. The direction of an impulse can be expressed by the number of degrees clockwise (positive) or anti clockwise (negative) of lead I, which is the zero reference point. For example, an impulse towards lead aVL has an axis of –30 degrees and an impulse towards lead III has an axis of +120 degrees (Figure 4.4).

Mean frontal QRS axis

The mean frontal QRS axis describes the dominant or average direction of the various electrical forces that develop during ventricular activation. Normally, the mean frontal QRS axis lies between aVL (i.e. –30 degrees) and aVF (i.e. +90 degrees).

If the axis is counter-clockwise, or to the left of aVL (i.e. less than –30 degrees), it is termed abnormal left axis deviation. If the axis is clockwise, or to the right of aVF (i.e. more than +90 degrees), there is right axis deviation.

Using the hexaxial reference system, the mean frontal QRS axis may be calculated to within a few degrees. However, this degree of precision is unnecessary. It is easier to diagnose left and right axis deviation from a simple rule of thumb, as follows.

In left axis deviation, lead I is mainly positive and *both* leads II and III are mainly negative (Figure 4.5). Contrary to some older texts, both II and III must be mainly

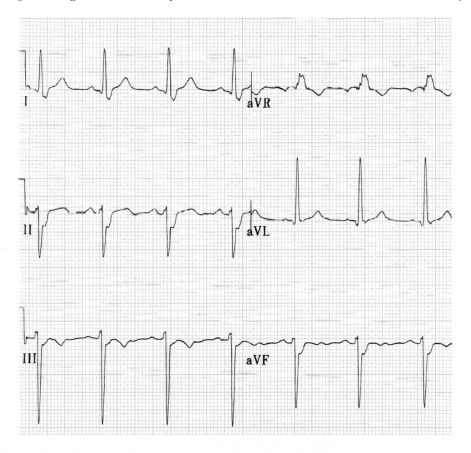

Figure 4.5 Left axis deviation due to left anterior fascicular block

negative, i.e. if in lead II the S wave is smaller than the R wave, abnormal left axis deviation is not present (Figure 4.6). If lead II is equiphasic, there is borderline left axis deviation (Figure 4.6).

In right axis deviation, lead I is mainly negative and both leads II and III are predominantly positive (Figure 4.7).

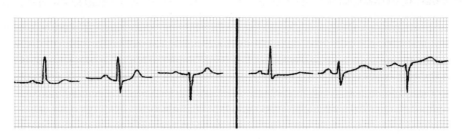

Figure 4.6 Leads I, II, III from two patients. In the first, the mean frontal QRS axis is normal. In the second, lead II is equiphasic and thus there is borderline left axis deviation

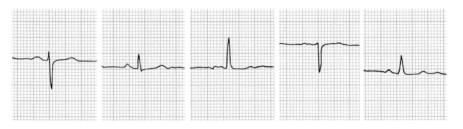

Figure 4.7 Right axis deviation due to left posterior fascicular block (leads I, II, III, aVL, aVF)

LEFT ANTERIOR FASCICULAR BLOCK

Block in the anterior fascicle of the left bundle branch causes delay in activation of the anterosuperior portion of the left ventricle. Initial left ventricular activation will be via the posterior fascicle to the posteroinferior region and will therefore be directed inferiorly and to the right. This results in an initial positive deflection (i.e. r wave) in inferiorly orientated leads (II, III and aVF) and in an initial negative deflection (i.e. q wave) in the lateral leads (I and aVL) (Figure 4.5).

The anterosuperior region will be activated by conduction from the postero-inferior region. The resultant wave will, therefore, be superiorly directed (R wave in I and aVL; S in II, III and aVF). Because conduction is through ordinary myocardium rather than the specialized conducting tissues, it will be relatively slow. As a result, activation of the anterosuperior region will be delayed and thus unopposed by activity from the rest of the ventricles. Thus the resultant superiorly directed wave is larger than the initial inferiorly directed wave and the mean frontal QRS axis will also be superiorly directed, i.e. there will be left axis deviation.

Left anterior fascicular block is a common cause of left axis deviation. The other cause is inferior myocardial infarction (Figure 4.8).

To diagnose left anterior fascicular block two criteria must be satisfied:

1. there must be left axis deviation, i.e. lead I must be predominantly positive and both leads II and III predominantly negative.
2. the initial direction of ventricular activation must be inferior and to the right, i.e. there must be an initial r wave in leads II, III and aVF.

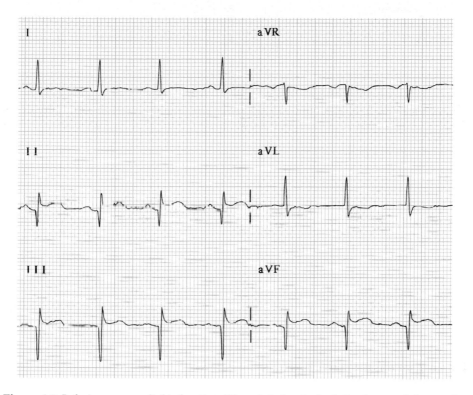

Figure 4.8 Inferior myocardial infarction. There is left axis deviation but not left anterior fascicular block

LEFT POSTERIOR FASCICULAR BLOCK

In left posterior fascicular block, activation of the posteroinferior portion of the left ventricle is delayed. As a result, there will be an initial positive r wave in leads I and aVL and an initial negative q wave in leads II, III and aVF; and there will be right axis deviation, i.e. lead I will be predominantly negative and leads II and III predominantly positive (Figure 4.7).

A diagnosis of left posterior fascicular block can only be made in the absence of other causes of right axis deviation such as right ventricular hypertrophy or strain, or a young patient with an asthenic build.

Main points

- Complete bundle branch block prolongs QRS duration to 0.12 s or greater. In incomplete block, QRS duration is 0.10–0.11 s.

- In abnormal left axis deviation, lead I is predominantly positive and both leads II and III are predominantly negative.

- In right axis deviation, lead I is predominantly negative and both leads II and III positive.

- The criteria for left anterior hemiblock are left axis deviation together with a small, initial r wave in leads II and aVF.

- Left posterior hemiblock should be considered when there is right axis deviation in the absence of its other causes, e.g. right ventricular hypertrophy or strain.

CHAPTER 5

The supraventricular tachycardias

MAIN TYPES

Several tachycardias originate from the atria or AV junction and are therefore, by definition, supraventricular in origin (Table 5.1). They have one thing in common: because they arise from above the level of the bundle branches, ventricular activation is via the rapidly conducting specialized intraventricular system and thus normal, and therefore narrow, ventricular complexes will usually result. However, it is very important to appreciate there are significant differences in mechanism, ECG characteristic and treatment. It is necessary to identify the type of tachycardia and not merely treat all tachycardias with narrow QRS complexes as 'supraventricular tachycardia'.

Table 5.1 Supraventricular tachycardias

1.	Atrioventricular re-entrant tachycardia
2.	Atrioventricular nodal re-entrant tachycardia
3.	Atrial fibrillation
4.	Atrial flutter
5.	Atrial tachycardia
6.	Sinus tachycardia (see chapter 1)

ATRIAL ORIGIN VERSUS ATRIOVENTRICULAR RE-ENTRY

Supraventricular tachycardia can be caused by two main mechanisms.

First, there are the re-entrant tachycardias (*see* chapter 9). There is an additional electrical connection between atria and ventricles, so an impulse can repeatedly and rapidly circulate between atria and ventricles along a circuit consisting of the AV junction and the additional AV connection.

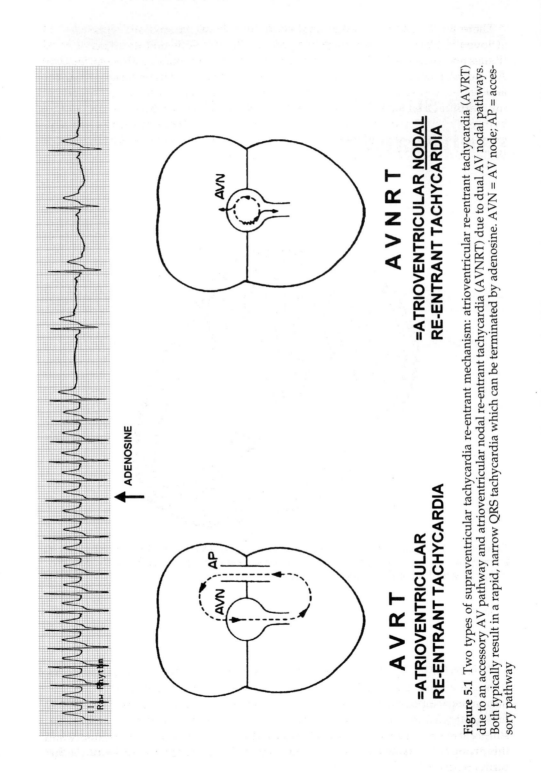

Figure 5.1 Two types of supraventricular tachycardia re-entrant mechanism: atrioventricular re-entrant tachycardia (AVRT) due to an accessory AV pathway and atrioventricular nodal re-entrant tachycardia (AVNRT) due to dual AV nodal pathways. Both typically result in a rapid, narrow QRS tachycardia which can be terminated by adenosine. AVN = AV node; AP = accessory pathway

Within the image:

Raw Rhythm

ADENOSINE

AVRT

=ATRIOVENTRICULAR
RE-ENTRANT TACHYCARDIA

AP

AVN

AVNRT

=ATRIOVENTRICULAR NODAL
RE-ENTRANT TACHYCARDIA

AVN

There are two types of additional connection between atria and ventricles. In atrioventricular nodal re-entrant tachycardia, the AV node and its adjacent atrial tissues are functionally dissociated into fast and slow AV nodal pathways, i.e. dual AV nodal pathways (Figure 5.1). In atrioventricular re-entrant tachycardia, the additional connection is an accessory AV pathway, which is a strand of myocardium that straddles the groove between atria and ventricles and therefore bypasses the AV node (Figure 5.2). If the accessory AV pathway can conduct antero-gradely, i.e. from atria to ventricles, then the patient will have the features of the Wolff–Parkinson–White syndrome (*see* chapter 10).

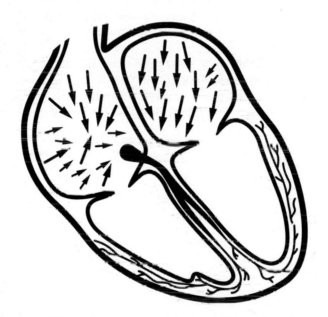

Figure 5.2 Diagram illustrating supraventricular tachycardias due to rapid atrial activity which is conducted to the ventricles via the AV node but the node is not an integral part of the arrhythmia mechanism

The second group of supraventricular tachycardias comprises those caused by rapid, abnormal atrial activity, i.e atrial tachycardia, flutter and fibrillation. The mechanism responsible for the tachycardia is confined to the atria. In contrast to the first group, the AV node is not an integral part of the tachycardia mechanism but simply transmits some or all the atrial impulses to the ventricles. Arrhythmias in this group are atrial fibrillation (chapter 6), atrial flutter (chapter 7) and atrial tachy-cardia (chapter 8).

SYMPTOMS CAUSED BY SUPRAVENTRICULAR TACHYCARDIAS

Paroxysmal supraventricular tahycardias may cause major symptoms: syncope or near-syncope, particularly at the onset of the arrhythmia; distressing palpitation; angina, even in the absence of coronary artery disease; dyspnoea; fatigue and polyuria. Other patients will merely be aware of but not distressed by palpitation or may even be asymptomatic.

Patients can be distressed not only by the symptoms caused by their tachycardia but also by the unpredictable nature of the arrhythmia. They may be frightened to travel or even to go out – for fear that a tachycardia might occur. Many patients do not have structural heart disease but they fear that the arrhythmia is a sign of impending heart attack or other major cardiac catastrophe. They need to be reassured that they have an 'electrical' rather than 'plumbing' or structural problem.

Supraventricular arrhythmias, if sustained, especially atrial tachycardia, atrioventricular re-entrant tachycardia (AVRT), and atrial fibrillation with a very rapid ventricular response, can lead to heart failure. The term 'tachy-cardiomyopathy' is applied. Restoration of normal rhythm will reverse the failure (Figure 5.3).

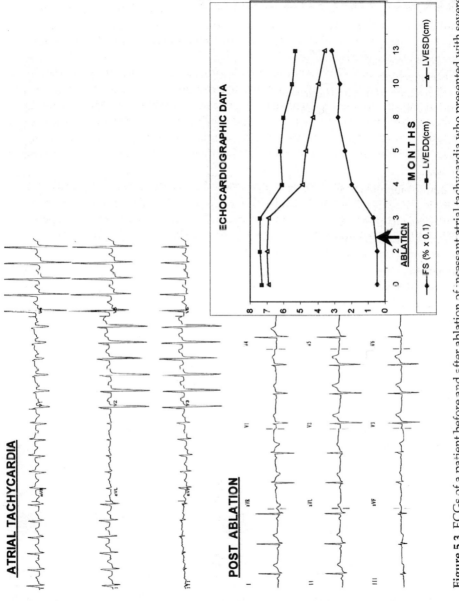

Figure 5.3 ECGs of a patient before and after ablation of incessant atrial tachycardia who presented with severe heart failure. Over the months, left ventricular end-diastolic (LVEDD) and end-systolic (LVESD) dimensions and fractional shortening (FS) returned to normal

Atrial fibrillation

This is the most common of all cardiac arrhythmias and it is important to be familiar with the causes, clinical manifestations and treatments of this heart rhythm disturbance.

During atrial fibrillation, the atria discharge at a rate of between 350 and 600 beats/min. The arrhythmia is due to multiple wavelets of electrical activity randomly circulating within the atrial myocardium.

ECG CHARACTERISTICS

ATRIAL ACTIVITY

The rapid and chaotic atrial activity during atrial fibrillation results in small, irregular waves at a rate of 350–600 beats/min. The amplitude of these 'f' waves varies from patient to patient, and also from ECG lead to lead: in some leads, 'f' waves may not be apparent, whereas in other leads, especially lead V1, the waves may appear so coarse that atrial flutter is suspected (Figures 6.1 and 6.2).

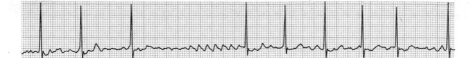

Figure 6.1 Typical 'f' waves of atrial fibrillation

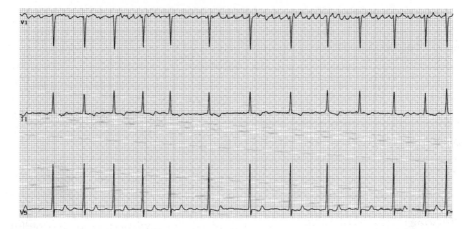

Figure 6.2 Atrial fibrillation. 'f' waves appear coarse in V1, fine in II and are not seen in V5. There is a totally irregular ventricular rhythm

ATRIOVENTRICULAR CONDUCTION

Fortunately, the atrioventricular node cannot conduct every atrial impulse to the ventricles. Some are totally blocked. Others only partially penetrate the atrioventricular node. They will not therefore activate the ventricles but may block or delay succeeding impulses. This process of 'concealed conduction' is responsible for **the totally irregular ventricular rhythm which is the hallmark of this arrhythmia.** In the absence of P waves, even if 'f' waves are not seen, a totally irregular ventricular rhythm is diagnostic of atrial fibrillation. Atrial fibrillation with a rapid ventricular rhythm is often misdiagnosed. If the characteristic irregular rhythm is remembered, errors will not be made (Figure 6.3). If, however, there is complete atrioventricular block, ventricular activity will, of course, be slow and regular (Figure 6.4).

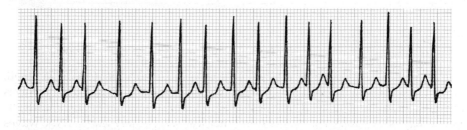

Figure 6.3 Atrial fibrillation with rapid ventricular response

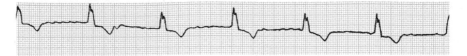

Figure 6.4 Atrial fibrillation with complete AV block. The ventricular rhythm is regular

The ventricular rate during atrial fibrillation is dependent on the conducting ability of the AV node which is itself influenced by the autonomic nervous system. Atrioventricular conduction will be enhanced by sympathetic activity and depressed by high vagal tone. In patients with normal atrioventricular conduction, the ventricular rate ranges from 100 to 200 beats/min.

INTRAVENTRICULAR CONDUCTION

Ventricular complexes during atrial fibrillation are of normal duration unless there is established bundle branch block, Wolff–Parkinson–White syndrome (discussed below) or aberrant intraventricular conduction.

Aberrant conduction is the result of unequal recovery periods of the bundle branches. An early atrial impulse may reach the ventricles when one bundle branch is still refractory to excitation following the previous cardiac cycle but the other is capable of conduction. The resultant ventricular complex will have a bundle branch block configuration. Because the right bundle usually has the longer refractory period, aberrant conduction commonly leads to right bundle branch block. The duration of the refractory period is related to the preceding cycle length. Thus, aberration is likely to occur when a short cycle succeeds a long cycle (Figure 6.5).

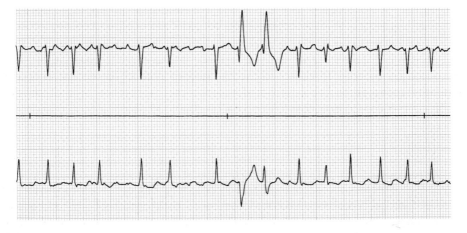

Figure 6.5 Atrial fibrillation. After seven normally conducted ventricular complexes, there are two complexes with right bundle branch block configuration

INITIATION

Atrial fibrillation is usually initiated by an atrial extrasystole (Figure 6.6). Sometimes atrial flutter or atrioventricular re-entrant tachycardia degenerate into atrial fibrillation.

Table 6.1 Characteristics of atrial fibrillation

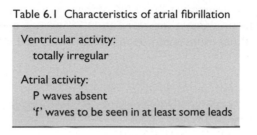

Ventricular activity:
  totally irregular

Atrial activity:
  P waves absent
  'f' waves to be seen in at least some leads

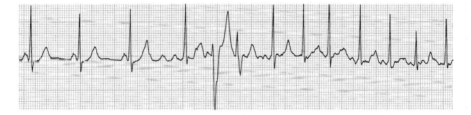

Figure 6.6 Atrial ectopic beat superimposed on T wave of third sinus beat initiates atrial fibrillation. Second and third complexes during atrial fibrillation are aberrantly conducted

CAUSES

The main causes are heart muscle damage due to coronary artery disease, hypertension or cardiomyopathy; rheumatic heart valve disease; hyperthyroidism; sick sinus syndrome; hypertrophic cardiomyopathy; thoracotomy, especially coronary bypass surgery; chronic obstructive airways disease; acute or chronic alcohol abuse; and constrictive pericarditis. Rarely, the arrhythmia is familial. In a substantial proportion of cases, atrial fibrillation is idiopathic, i.e. there is no demonstrable cause.

Coronary artery disease *per se* does not cause atrial fibrillation. However, the arrhythmia often results from myocardial infarction, both acutely and in the long term, and is an indicator of extensive myocardial damage.

A cause for atrial fibrillation should always be sought. Many of the causes can be identified or excluded by clinical examination, electrocardiography and echocardiography. Measurement of serum thyroxine is often necessary to exclude hyperthyroidism. Ambulatory electrocardiography may be required where sick sinus syndrome is a possibility.

PREVALENCE

Prevalence increases with age. In a survey of male civil servants in the United Kingdom, atrial fibrillation was found in 0.16%, 0.37% and 1.13% of those aged 40–49 years, 50–59 years and 60–64 years, respectively. A total of 3.7% of patients over 65 years in a British general practice were found to have the arrhythmia. The Framingham study demonstrated that 7.8% of men between aged 65–74 years had atrial fibrillation. The prevalence increased to 11.7% in men aged 75–84 years. The arrhythmia was 1.5 times more common in men than women.

PROGNOSIS

One of the major determinants of prognosis is the presence or absence of organic heart disease. For example, in patients with coronary artery disease, because atrial fibrillation is usually a result of extensive myocardial damage, it indicates a poor prognosis. Most studies have shown that idiopathic atrial fibrillation has a very good prognosis.

SYSTEMIC EMBOLISM

During atrial fibrillation, stasis of blood in the left atrium can lead to thrombus formation and systemic embolism. Of particular concern is the risk of stroke. The echocardiographic signs of left atrial stasis are spontaneous echo contrast and reduced left atrial appendage flow velocity.

Increased levels of plasma fibrinogen and fibrin D-dimer have been found in atrial fibrillation. Levels return to normal after cardioversion suggesting that it may be atrial fibrillation itself which causes a 'hypercoagulable' state.

Risk

Atrial fibrillation caused by rheumatic mitral valve disease leads to a very high (15-fold) risk of stroke. 'Nonrheumatic' causes of atrial fibrillation, mainly congestive cardiac failure and hypertension, are associated with a moderately high (five-fold) risk of embolism with an incidence of approximately 5% per annum. Furthermore, computerized tomography has demonstrated a 14% incidence of asymptomatic cerebral infarction in these patients.

The risk of embolism in non-rheumatic atrial fibrillation increases with age: it is small in those less than 60 years.

Embolism is rare in idiopathic atrial fibrillation: less than 1% per annum.

ANTICOAGULATION

Warfarin markedly reduces the risk of embolism but at a small increased risk of intracranial haemorrhage and other forms of bleeding. Studies have shown that very low dose warfarin is ineffective and have indicated that the ideal international normalized ratio (INR) of the prothrombin time is 2.5.

Based on current information, all patients with rheumatic heart disease, and those with non-rheumatic atrial fibrillation who are at high risk (e.g. history of embolism, over 60 years of age, evidence of coronary disease, myocardial dysfunction, diabetes or left atrial enlargement) who can cope with and who have no contra-indications to anticoagulation, should receive warfarin.

Aspirin is a more convenient alternative to warfarin for many patients but studies indicate that it is less effective. It is, however, likely that some patients with non-rheumatic atrial fibrillation are at risk from stroke from causes other than the left atrial thrombus: for example, patients with myocardial damage caused by coronary disease may also have carotid artery stenosis. Atrial fibrillation in these patients may be a 'marker' of vascular disease; aspirin (300 mg daily) may well be beneficial in them.

IDIOPATHIC ATRIAL FIBRILLATION

Idiopathic or 'lone' atrial fibrillation is a common problem. While the prognosis is good and the risk of systemic embolism is low, lone atrial fibrillation can cause very troublesome symptoms and great anxiety. Like secondary atrial fibrillation, it may be paroxysmal or, less commonly, persistent.

PAROXYSMAL LONE ATRIAL FIBRILLATION

Some patients will experience only a single or a very occasional episode. Others will experience frequent recurrences, perhaps several times in a day. Paroxysms may last for many hours or stop after only a few seconds (Figure 6.7).

Some patients will suffer major symptoms. Others, including some with frequent attacks and rapid ventricular rates, will be asymptomatic or merely aware of but not distressed by palpitation.

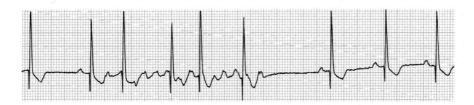

Figure 6.7 A brief episode of atrial fibrillation

In a minority of patients there will be an identifiable precipitating event such as exercise, vomiting, overindulgence in alcohol, or fatigue. One form of paroxysmal lone atrial fibrillation has been attributed to high vagal activity: the arrhythmia always starts at rest, during bradycardia, and can be initiated by manoeuvres that increase vagal tone (Figure 6.8) .

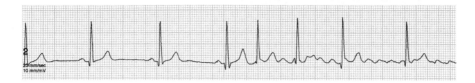

Figure 6.8 Onset of atrial fibrillation at rest during sinus rate 50 beats/min

TREATMENT

The choice of treatment depends on whether the purpose is to control the ventricular response to atrial fibrillation or to maintain sinus rhythm, a decision which will be influenced by the cause and duration of the arrhythmia.

Treatment of persistent atrial fibrillation is usually aimed at preventing a fast ventricular rate by a drug or drugs which depress atrioventricular nodal conduction. Though drugs frequently effect a return to sinus rhythm when the arrhythmia is of recent onset, they are otherwise rarely successful. Cardioversion can usually restore sinus rhythm but atrial fibrillation often recurs.

In paroxysmal atrial fibrillation, oral anti-arrhythmic drugs will often prevent a recurrence.

CONTROL OF VENTRICULAR RESPONSE TO ATRIAL FIBRILLATION

Digoxin

Oral digoxin provides effective long-term control of persistent atrial fibrillation in many patients and remains the drug of first choice. It has the advantages that it has a long duration of action and is not negatively inotropic. However, digoxin sometimes fails to control the heart rate at rest and is often ineffective at controlling the rate during exertion in spite of high serum concentrations.

Given intravenously, digoxin is often ineffective at promptly reducing the ventricular response to atrial fibrillation.

Calcium antagonists

Intravenous verapamil quickly and effectively depresses atrioventricular conduction and will thereby control a rapid ventricular response to atrial fibrillation within a few minutes. However, it is unlikely to restore sinus rhythm and indeed there is some evidence to suggest that verapamil will encourage the arrhythmia to persist.

When digoxin alone is inadequate, the addition of oral verapamil (40–80 mg t.d.s.) is extremely effective in controlling the ventricular rate during atrial fibrillation, both at rest and on exertion. Verapamil increases serum digoxin concentrations but this mechanism is not thought to be responsible for its beneficial effect. Verapamil alone may be effective but is not superior to digoxin.

Diltiazem (but not nifedipine or amlodipine) has similar actions to verapamil.

Beta-blockers

Beta-blocking drugs will also slow the heart rate during atrial fibrillation in digitalized patients but may be contraindicated if myocardial function is severely impaired.

Fast and slow ventricular rates

Some patients demonstrate very fast and slow ventricular responses to atrial fibrillation. Ventricular pacing may be required to allow introduction of AV nodal-blocking drugs (Figures 6.9 and 6.10).

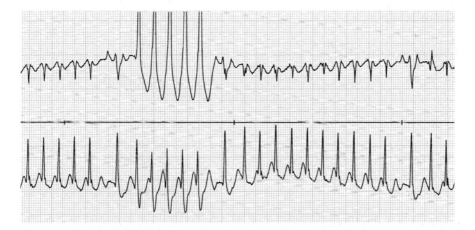

Figure 6.9 Very fast ventricular respone to atrial fibrillation. Aberrant conduction of seventh to eleventh ventricular complexes.

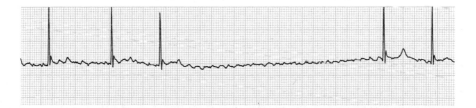

Figure 6.10 Very slow ventricular response during the night in the same patient as in Figure 6.9

RESTORATION OF SINUS RHYTHM

Restoration and maintenance of sinus rhythm, if possible, is preferable to control of the ventricular response to atrial fibrillation. The advantages are haemodynamic improvement, reduction in risk of systemic embolism and avoidance of the unwanted effects from anti-arrhythmic drugs.

Anti-arrhythmic drugs

It should be borne in mind that approximately half of episodes of recent onset atrial fibrillation will terminate spontaneously within 8 h.

Intravenous flecainide, propafenone, sotalol and amiodarone may restore normal rhythm (i.e. achieve chemical cardioversion) provided atrial fibrillation is of recent onset. However, these drugs, particularly flecainide, can sometimes fail to restore normal rhythm but slow the atrial rate, and thus convert atrial fibrillation to atrial flutter or tachycardia. Paradoxically, the lower atrial rate can lead to a marked acceleration of the ventricular rate because the AV node can conduct a greater proportion of atrial impulses – occasionally necessitating prompt electrical cardioversion.

Digoxin is unlikely to restore sinus rhythm and there is evidence to show that it may actually help perpetuate the arrhythmia by shortening the refractory period of atrial myocardium.

Electrical cardioversion

Sinus rhythm can be restored by electrical cardioversion in most patients with atrial fibrillation. However, the arrhythmia frequently returns. Only a third of patients will remain in normal rhythm in the long term.

High-energy shocks are often required for successful cardioversion of atrial fibrillation (*see* chapter 20). Drugs such as flecainide, sotalol, disopyramide, propafenone and amiodarone reduce the relapse rate after cardioversion. The latter has been shown to be the most effective.

Cardioversion can result in immediate systemic embolism because of dislodgement of pre-existing thrombus. New atrial thrombus can develop after cardioversion because atrial mechanical activity often does not return for up to 3 weeks after the procedure and because cardioversion itself can increase blood hypercoagulabilty. Hence embolism can also occur in the following few weeks. It is therefore recommended that non-urgent cardioversion in patients who have been in atrial fibrillation for more than 24 h is preceded by warfarin for at least 3 weeks and that anticoagulation is continued for 4 weeks after restoration of normal rhythm. If cardioversion has to be carried out urgently it should be preceded by heparin.

While cardioversion only leads to long-term sinus rhythm in a minority of patients, an attempt at restoring sinus rhythm should be considered in those patients with recent atrial fibrillation (less than 12 months) where no cause has been identified or in whom the disorder which has caused the arrhythmia has resolved or is self-limiting. If there is a recurrence, a further attempt at cardioversion, after initiation of anti-arrhythmic therapy, should be undertaken in those with troublesome symptoms attributable to the arrhythmia.

There are reports of successful cardioversion in patients with atrial fibrillation which has persisted in excess of 12–24 months. In patients with atrial fibrillation which is dificult to treat, even if long-standing, cardioversion should also be considered because there is a small chance that normal rhythm will be achieved and maintained.

Recently, transvenous cardioversion has been introduced. A low-energy shock is delivered between transvenous electrodes positioned in the right atrium and either the coronary sinus or pulmonary artery. Higher success rates than for transthoracic cardioversion, especially in very large patients, have been reported.

Prevention of recurrence of paroxysmal atrial fibrillation

Trial and error is often necessary to find a drug which is both effective and well tolerated. Sotalol, flecainide, disopyramide and propafenone may be effective. In patients where the arrhythmia usually starts when the patient is active, sotalol is the preferred drug while, if atrial fibrillation usually occurs at rest, Class I drugs such as flecainide are preferable.

Quinidine had been used for many years to prevent paroxysmal atrial fibrillation. However, a meta-analysis of studies of the efficacy of quinidine in preventing recurrence of atrial fibrillation found that the drug was associated with a significant increase in mortality, presumably due to a pro-arrhythmic effect.

Digoxin shortens the atrial refractory period and may thereby increase the tendency to atrial fibrillation. There is no evidence that it prevents the arrhythmia or slows the ventricular rate during an acute episode. Digoxin should not be used in paroxysmal atrial fibrillation.

'Refractory' atrial fibrillation

Amiodarone is a very potent anti-arrhythmic drug which will often maintain sinus rhythm or at least control the ventricular response to atrial fibrillation when other drugs have failed. However, in view of the high incidence of major unwanted effects, the drug should be reserved for patients in whom other drugs have failed and for patients in whom the risk of side-effects in the long term may not be a major consideration because their prognosis is poor, e.g. the elderly and those with severe myocardial damage.

Transvenous radiofrequency ablation of the atrioventricular junction should be considered in patients in whom anti-arrhythmic drugs are ineffective or cannot be tolerated (see Chapter 26). It necessitates pacemaker implantation and in many cases oral anticoagulation, but it is very effective at controlling symptoms and has been demonstrated in several studies to improve patients' quality of life. It also avoids the need for anti-arrhythmic therapy.

Recently, radiofrequency ablation has been shown to be effective in preventing paroxysmal atrial fibrillation. It is necessary to deliver radiofrequency energy to the site of origin of the atrial ectopic beats which initiate the arrhythmia. The commonset sites of origin have been shown to be in one or more of the pulmonary veins. However, in contrast to ablation of the AV node, the procedure currently is of limited efficacy, time consuming and involves significant risks, namely, stroke and pulmonary vein thrombosis.

An implantable atrial defibrillator has become available for the control of paroxysmal atrial fibrillation. The device is usually activated by the patient rather than discharging a shock automatically. Shock delivery is painful and, clearly, the device is only suitable for patients with infrequent episodes. Apart from pain, concerns include the unpredictable nature of paroxysmal atrial fibrillation and the high rate of early or even immediate recurrence of the arrhythmia. For these reasons implantation rates are low and the explantation rate is substantial.

There is increasing interest in atrial pacing to prevent paroxysmal atrial fibrillation. Stimulation of the atrial septum or simultaneous stimulation of the right atrial appendage and coronary os have been shown to abbbreviate the duration of atrial activation – an important determinant of predisposition to paroxysmal atrial fibrillation. Studies have shown that, in some patients, the arrhythmia can be prevented by these pacing modes, though, in the author's experience, it is usually necessary to continue an anti-arrhythmic drug such as flecainide that without pacing was ineffective.

Main points

- Atrial fibrillation is characterized by a totally irregular ventricular rhythm and absence of P waves. The chaotic atrial activity results in rapid, small, irregular 'f' waves which many not be seen in all ECG leads.

- The main causes are heart muscle damage from ischaemia or cardio-myopathy, rheumatic heart valve disease, hyperthyroidism, sick sinus syndrome, thoracotomy, obstructive airways disease and alcohol abuse. Often, atrial fibrillation is idiopathic.

- Prevalence increases with age.

- The arrhythmia may be paroxysmal or persistent.

- Sotalol, flecainide and amiodarone may prevent paroxysmal atrial fibrillation. Digoxin is of no use.

- Although cardioversion usually restores sinus rhythm, there is a high relapse rate. High-energy shocks are required.

- AV nodal-blocking drugs are used to control the ventricular response to persistent atrial fibrillation. Digoxin may fail to control the rate during exercise.

- Atrial fibrillation may cause systemic embolism which can be prevented by warfarin. Rheumatic mitral valve disease leads to a very high risk of stroke. 'Nonrheumatic' causes of atrial fibrillation are associated with a moderately high risk. The risk in nonrheumatic atrial fibrillation increases with age: it is small in those less than 60 years. Embolism is rare in idiopathic atrial fibrillation.

Atrial flutter

In the typical form of atrial flutter, the atria discharge at a rate between 240 and 350 beats/min. Usually, the atrial rate is close to 300 beats/min. The arrhythmia is caused by a re-entrant circuit within the right atrium. Usually, the impulse circulates in an inferior direction along the lateral border of the right atrium and returns in a superior direction along the inter-atrial septum (Figure 7.1).

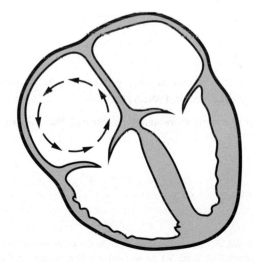

Figure 7.1 Common atrial flutter: counterclockwise circuit within the right atrium

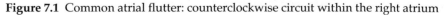

ECG CHARACTERISTICS

Atrial flutter may be paroxysmal or sustained. It is usually initiated by an atrial extrasystole. It may degenerate into atrial fibrillation.

ATRIAL ACTIVITY

During the typical form of atrial flutter, the atria discharge regularly at a rate of approximately 300 beats/min. In many leads there will be no isoelectric line between atrial deflections or 'F' waves, leading to the characteristic sawtooth appearance which is usually best seen in leads II, III, and aVF. However, in some leads, especially lead V1, atrial activity will be seen in the form of discrete waves (Figure 7.2).

Commonly in typical atrial flutter, the atrial impulse circulates counterclockwise within the right atrium in which case the 'F' waves are negative in leads II, III and aVF, of very low amplitude in lead I and positive in V1 (Figure 7.2). Uncommonly, the impulse circulates in a clockwise direction (Figure 7.3).

In atypical atrial flutter, the atrial rate is faster, ranging from 350 to 450 beats/min; F waves are positive in the inferior leads.

ATRIOVENTRICULAR CONDUCTION

As with atrial fibrillation, the ventricular response to atrial flutter is determined by the conducting ability of the atrioventricular junction. Most commonly, alternate 'F'

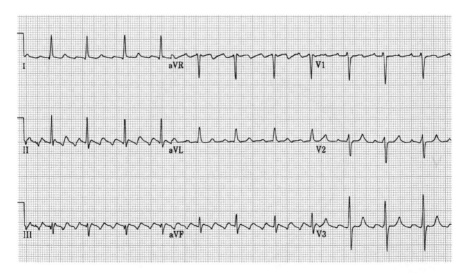

Figure 7.2 Typical atrial flutter: negative sawtooth pattern in the inferior leads and positive, discrete F waves in lead V1 as is seen in the common form of typical atrial flutter

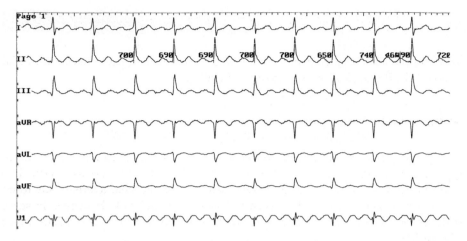

Figure 7.3 Uncommon form of typical atrial flutter due to clockwise rotation within the right atrial re-entrant circuit

waves are conducted to the ventricles with a resultant ventricular rate of close to 150 beats/min (Figure 7.4). Drugs or impaired atrioventricular nodal function may lead to a higher degree of atrioventricular block (Figure 7.5) . High levels of sympathetic nervous system activity, as may occur during exercise, may enhance atrioventricular nodal conduction and result in 1:1 conduction and a ventricular rate of approximately 300 beats/min (Figure 7.6).

With high degrees of atrioventricular block, atrial activity is clearly discernible and the arrhythmia is easy to diagnose (Figure 7.7). However, during a rapid ventricular response, ventricular T waves may be superimposed on alternate 'F'

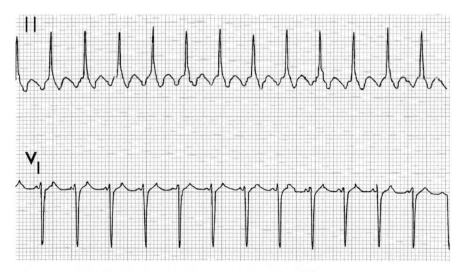

Figure 7.4 Atrial flutter with 2:1 AV block. Lead II shows a classic sawtooth appearance while V1 shows discrete atrial waves. In V1 each QRS complex is immediately preceded by an F wave and is followed by an F wave which is superimposed on the T wave

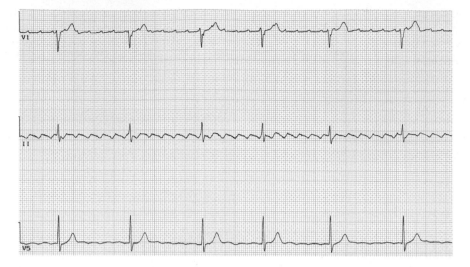

Figure 7.5 Atrial flutter with slow ventricular response

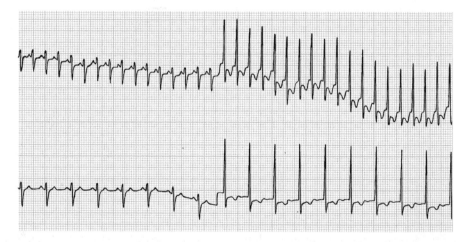

Figure 7.6 Continuous recordings of leads V1 and V4. In the upper trace the ventricular rate is 300 beats/min, suggesting atrial flutter with 1:1 AV conduction. The lower trace shows the effect of carotid massage. The ventricular rate is halved and F waves can be seen in V1 immediately before the QRS complex and superimposed on the T wave

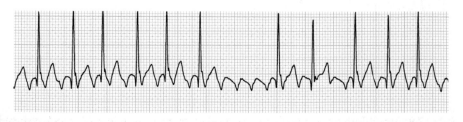

Figure 7.7 Atrial flutter only clearly seen during transient increase in AV block

waves and may obscure the characteristic atrial activity: sinus tachycardia may be mistakenly diagnosed (Figure 7.8). Atrial flutter should be suspected if the heart rate is 150 beats/min at rest. Carotid sinus massage or adenosine can transiently impair atrioventricular conduction and aid diagnosis (Figure 7.9).

INTRAVENTRICULAR CONDUCTION

Ventricular complexes will be normal in duration unless there is bundle branch block, ventricular pre-excitation or aberrant intraventricular conduction.

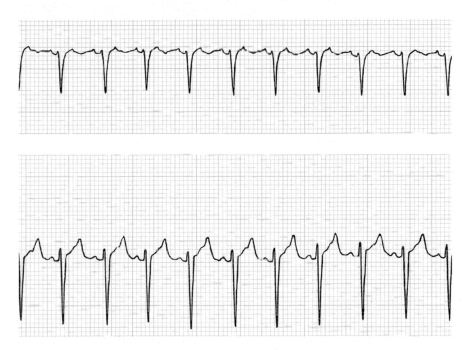

Figure 7.8 Simultaneous recording of leads V1 and V2. Atrial flutter can be diagnosed from V1 (alternate F waves are superimposed on the beginning of the ventricular T wave) but V2 looks like sinus tachycardia

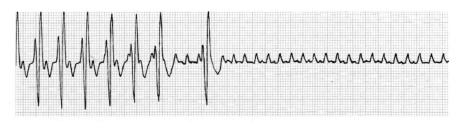

Figure 7.9 Atrial flutter revealed during several seconds of complete AV block induced by adenosine

Table 7.1 The characteristics of atrial flutter

Atrial activity:
'F' waves at rate of 300 beats/min
  'Sawtooth' appearance in limb leads
  Discrete atrial waves in VI

Ventricular activity:
  Rarely, 1:1 AV conduction resulting in ventricular rate of 300 beats/min
  Usually, 2:1 or higher degrees of AV block

CAUSES

Atrial flutter has similar aetiologies to atrial fibrillation, including idiopathic.

PREVALENCE

Atrial flutter is less common than atrial fibrillation. A recent survey reports an annual incidence of 88 per 100 000.

TREATMENT

Attempts to control a rapid ventricular response to atrial flutter by drugs are often unsuccessful. Where possible, the aim should be to restore and maintain sinus rhythm.

RESTORATION OF NORMAL RHYTHM

Cardioversion

Sustained atrial flutter can almost always be terminated with a low-energy DC shock, e.g. 50 joules (J). In the long term, atrial flutter will return in half of cases and further cardioversion or alternative treatment will be required.

The consensus is that, where possible, cardioversion should be preceded by anti-coagulation as for atrial fibrillation.

Anti-arrhythmic drugs

Drugs such as sotalol, flecainide, disopyramide and propafenone may be effective in terminating atrial flutter. However, it should be borne in mind that these drugs, if unsuccessful in restoring sinus rhythm, may possibly lead to higher ventricular rates. First, some drugs, particularly disopyramide, have a vagolytic effect which might enhance conduction through the atrioventricular node. Secondly, drugs often slow the atrial rate facilitating a reduction in the atrioventricular conduction ratio (*see* Figure 19.1). Ibutilide may be effective but may cause torsade de pointes tachycardia.

Rapid atrial pacing

Rapid atrial pacing at a rate approximately 25% in excess of the atrial rate (not the ventricular rate!) for 30–60 s will often restore sinus rhythm. Atrial fibrillation may sometimes be precipitated but usually sinus rhythm will return within a few hours.

Pacing is generally carried out transvenously. Stimulation of the low right atrium is more likely to lead to successful termination of the arrhythmia. It is important to ensure that pacing stimuli do capture the atria: capture is usually reflected in a change in the ventricular rate. The transoesophageal approach is favoured by some.

CONTROL OF VENTRICULAR RESPONSE

If normal rhythm cannot be restored or maintained, atrioventricular nodal-blocking drugs may be required to control a rapid ventricular response to atrial flutter. Intravenous verapamil or diltiazem will promptly slow the ventricular rate during atrial flutter. Oral digoxin and/or a calcium antagonist or beta-blocking drug can be employed as with atrial fibrillation. Sometimes, it is not possible to control the ventricular rate with oral drugs.

MAINTENANCE OF SINUS RHYTHM

Drugs which may prevent a recurrence of atrial fibrillation, as discussed above, are equally effective in preventing recurrence of atrial flutter.

'REFRACTORY' ATRIAL FLUTTER

Amiodarone can be very effective in maintaining sinus rhythm when other drugs have failed. Even if atrial flutter persists, the drug's actions in both slowing the atrial rate and depressing atrioventricular conduction can lead to a substantial slowing of the ventricular rate.

Radiofrequency ablation can be used to interrupt the re-entrant circuit in the right atrium and thereby prevent atrial flutter. Energy is usually delivered to the isthmus between the posterior portion of the tricuspid valve and the inferior vena cava. Success rates are not as high as in ablation of other arrhythmias but do compare favourably with anti-arrhythmic therapy. Atrial fibrillation can sometimes result in the longer term.

Transvenous ablation of the atrioventricular junction will achieve control of the ventricular rate but necessitates pacemaker implantation.

SYSTEMIC EMBOLISM

As with atrial fibrillation, atrial flutter can cause systemic embolism. Current evidence suggests that the risk is lower but patients with atrial flutter, who have clinical or echocardiographic findings that would indicate high risk if they had atrial fibrillation, should receive warfarin.

Main points

- The diagnosis of atrial flutter is based on the finding of atrial activity at a rate of approximately 300 beats/min.

- Usually atrial activity will be in the form of a sawtooth pattern in the limb leads but discrete 'F' waves will be seen in lead V1.

- Lead Vl is often the best lead for demonstrating atrial flutter: when there is 2:1 AV conduction, alternate 'F' waves will be superimposed on ventricular T waves.

- Where possible, a return to sinus rhythm should be sought.

- Cardioversion with low energy will usually terminate atrial flutter but there is a substantial recurrence rate, which may necessiate anti-arrhythmic therapy or radiofrequency ablation.

Atrial tachycardia

The practical difference between atrial tachycardia and flutter is that, in the former, the atrial rate is slower, being between 120 and 240 beats/min. Again, sometimes the AV node can conduct all atrial impulses but often there is a degree of AV block.

ECG CHARACTERISTICS

Because the atrial rate is slower, there is no sawtooth appearance to the baseline. Abnormally shaped P waves are inscribed at a regular rate (Figures 8.1 and 8.2). Usually, the ventricular complexes will be narrow unless there is pre-existent bundle branch block, or aberrant intraventricular conduction. Again like atrial flutter, atrial activity is often best seen in lead V1.

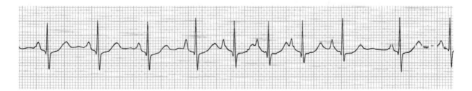

Figure 8.1 After three sinus beats, there is a short episode of atrial tachycardia: the rate abruptly increases and there is a change in P wave morphology

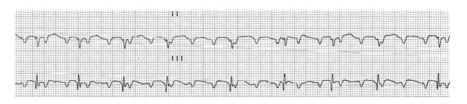

Figure 8.2 Atrial tachycardia with AV block. The atrial rate is 150 beats/min

Atrial tachycardia with 1:1 AV conduction may occur (Figure 8.3). As in atrial flutter, carotid sinus massage is often helpful in the diagnosis (Figure 8.4). However, it should be noted that, in some patients, adenosine will terminate atrial tachycardia without causing transient AV block.

A positive P wave in lead V1 points to a left atrial origin, while a positive P wave in lead aVL points to a right atrial origin.

With fairly high grades of AV block, because the atrial rate is relatively slow, the rhythm may be misdiagnosed as complete heart block and an inappropriate request made for cardiac pacing!

Atrial tachycardia is often paroxysmal. If incessant, however, it may lead to heart failure (*see* Figure 5.3).

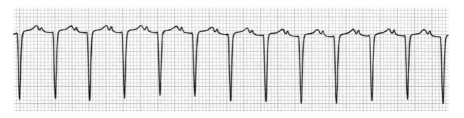

Figure 8.3 Lead V1. Atrial tachycardia with 1:1 AV conduction

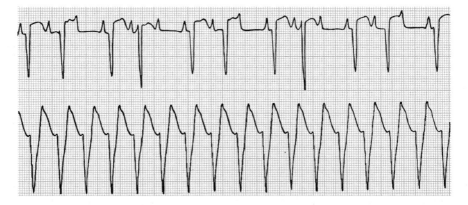

Figure 8.4 Lead V1. Atrial tachycardia before (lower trace) and during carotid sinus massage (upper trace). The atrial rate in the upper trace is the same as the ventricular rate in the lower trace, showing that without carotid massage there is 1:1 AV conduction

CAUSES

Causes include cardiomyopathy, chronic ischaemic heart disease, rheumatic heart disease, chronic obstructive airways disease and sick sinus syndrome. Not infrequently, no cause is found.

Atrial tachycardia with AV block may be due to digoxin toxicity (Figure 8.5). The arrhythmia is often referred to as 'paroxysmal atrial tachycardia with block', being

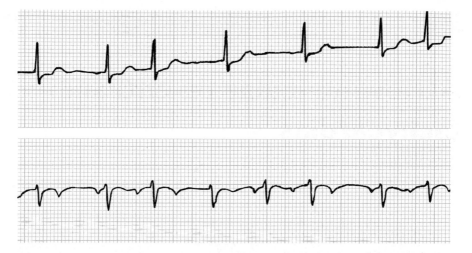

Figure 8.5 Atrial tachycardia (leads II and V1) in a patient with digoxin toxicity. Lead II suggests atrial fibrillation but V1 clearly shows atrial tachycardia with Mobitz I AV block

abbreviated to PATB. The term paroxysmal is inappropriate; particularly in the context of digoxin toxicity, the arrhythmia is usually sustained.

TREATMENT

- If the patient is receiving digoxin, toxicity should be suspected and the drug discontinued.
- If a return to sinus rhythm is required, cardioversion or rapid atrial pacing should be performed.
- Anti-arrhythmic drugs such as sotalol, flecainide and amiodarone may be effective.
- Radiofrequency ablation to the site of origin which is often in the lateral wall of the right atrium or near the pulmonary veins in the left atrium should be considered in refractory cases.

Main points

- The atrial rate is between 120 and 240 beats/min.
- The AV node may conduct all atrial impulses or there may be a degree of AV block.
- Carotid massage may aid diagnosis when there is doubt as to whether there is an atrial tachycardia.

Atrioventricular re-entrant tachycardias

In these supraventricular arrhythmias, as stated above, there is an additional connection between atria and ventricles so an impulse can repeatedly circulate along a circuit consisting of the AV junction and the additional AV connection. This is in contrast to the atrial arrhythmias discussed in the previous three chapters where the mechanism responsible for the tachycardia is confined to the atria and the AV node merely transmits some or all the atrial impulses to the ventricles.

MECHANISM

In most cases the heart is structurally normal, i.e. there is no valve, myocardial or coronary disease.

The impulse is usually conducted from atria to ventricles by the AV junction and then re-enters the atria via the additional connection (Figure 9.1).

The additional connection can be of one of the following two types.

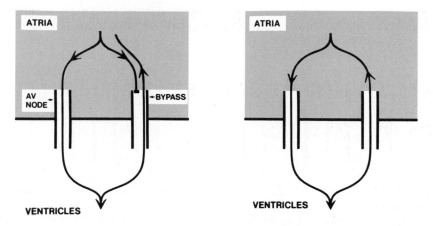

Figure 9.1 Initiation of AV re-entrant tachycardia. An atrial extrasystole arrives at the AV junction while the bypass tract is still refractory to excitation following the last cardiac cycle. The extrasystole is therefore only conducted to the ventricles via the AV node. By the time the extrasystole has traversed the AV node and reached the ventricles, the bypass tract has recovered and can conduct the impulse back to the atria (a), thereby initiating the re-entrant mechanism (b)

ACCESSORY AV PATHWAY

An accessory AV pathway is a strand of myocardium which straddles the groove between atria and ventricles and therefore bypasses the AV node. A re-entrant tachycardia involving an accessory AV pathway is termed an AV re-entrant tachycardia (AVRT).

DUAL AV NODAL PATHWAYS

The other type of additional connection occurs when the AV node and its adjacent atrial tissues are functionally dissociated into fast and slow AV nodal pathways, i.e. dual AV nodal pathways. Conduction from atria to ventricles is usually via a relatively slowly conducting AV nodal pathway while ventriculo-atrial conduction is via a fast AV pathway. A tachycardia due to dual AV nodal pathways is termed an AV nodal re-entrant tachycardia (AVNRT).

ECG CHARACTERISTICS

The tachycardia is regular and usually the QRS complexes are normal and therefore narrow (Figure 9.2). Occasionally pre-existing bundle branch block or bundle branch block caused by the tachycardia will lead to broad ventricular complexes (Figure 9.3).

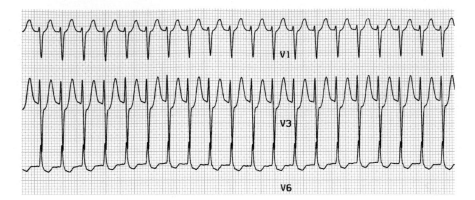

Figure 9.2 AV re-entrant tachycardia. A regular tachycardia with narrow ventricular complexes

The rate during tachycardia can range from 120 to 250 beats/min and is influenced by the sympathetic nervous system. For example, sympathetic activity and, consequently, the speed of AV nodal conduction increase on standing up so the tachycardia becomes faster.

Clearly, normal P waves will not occur during this arrhythmia. Since the circulating impulse re-enters the atria after ventricular activation, each QRS complex will be followed by a P wave, though this wave is not always detectable (Figures 9.4–9.6). If the atrial rate exceeds the ventricular rate, whether spontaneously or due to a drug or manoeuvre which slows AV node conduction, then the rhythm is not atrioventricular re-entrant tachycardia; it is probably atrial tachycardia or flutter.

ST segment and T wave changes can be caused by the tachycardia and persist for some time after its cessation; they are of no diagnostic significance.

The ECG during sinus rhythm is usually normal unless there is Wolff–Parkinson–White syndrome (*see* chapter 10).

TIMING OF ATRIAL ACTIVITY DURING TACHYCARDIA

The timing of atrial activity, if identifiable, may indicate whether the tachycardia is due to an accessory AV pathway, i.e. AV re-entry (AVRT), or due to dual AV nodal pathways, i.e. AV nodal re-entry (AVNRT). Distinction is relevant if the patient is a candidate for radiofrequency ablation.

With AVNRT, a P wave immediately follows or is superimposed on the QRS complex because the re-entrant circuit is small (Figures 9.4–9.6). The P wave is often best seen in lead V1. It might be mistaken for the secondary R wave of right bundle branch block but, if this were the case, the same wave should be present in lead V1 during sinus rhythm (Figures 9.5 and 9.6).

The length of the re-entrant circuit is greater in AVRT because the accessory AV pathway is some distance from the AV junction. It therefore takes longer for an

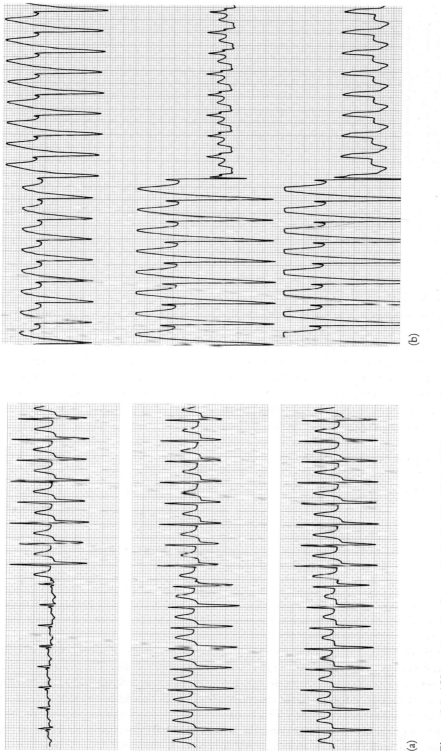

(a)

(b)

Figure 9.3 AV re-entrant tachycardia, leads V1–V6. (a) With narrow complexes. (b) A few minutes later, broad complexes have developed due to functional left bundle branch block

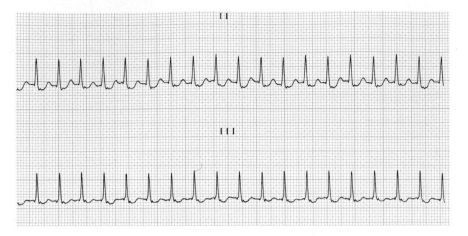

Figure 9.4 AV nodal re-entrant tachycardia. A small P wave immediately follows each QRS complex

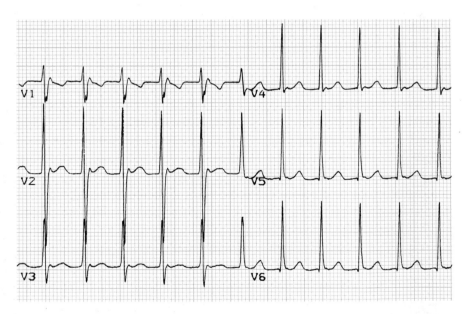

Figure 9.5 AV nodal re-entrant tachycardia. A small P wave can be seen after each QRS. In leads V1 and V2 it could be mistaken for a secondary R wave

impulse to circulate and re-enter the atria. Hence the inverted P wave occurs roughly halfway between QRS complexes and will therefore usually be super-imposed on the T wave (Figure 9.7). It can be identified because superimpostion of the P wave on the T wave usually leads to a pointed appearance of the T wave (Figures 9.8 and 9.9).

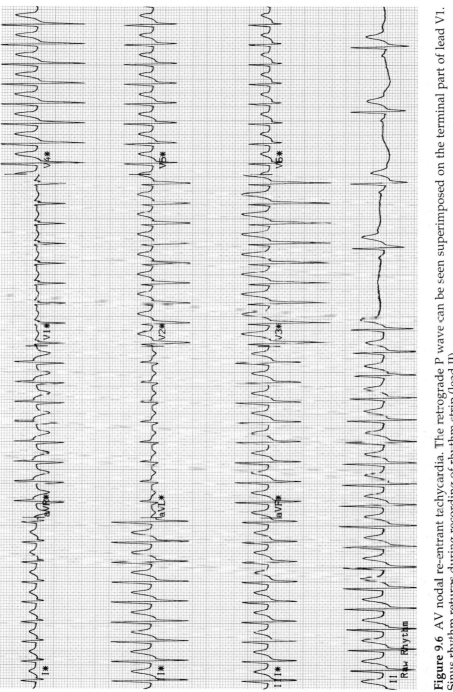

Figure 9.6 AV nodal re-entrant tachycardia. The retrograde P wave can be seen superimposed on the terminal part of lead V1. Sinus rhythm returns during recording of rhythm strip (lead II)

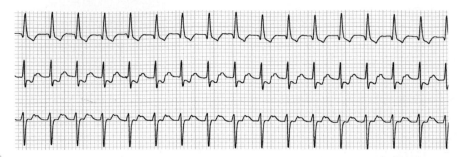

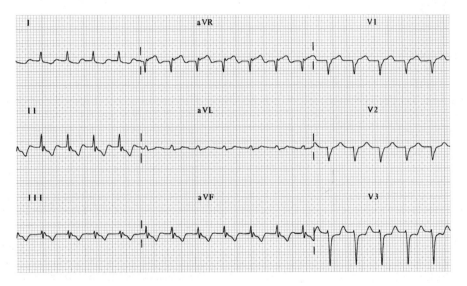

Figure 9.7 AV re-entrant tachycardia. There is a P wave after each QRS complex which is superimposed on the T wave, resulting in its pointed appearance. An inverted P wave in lead I suggests a left-sided accessory pathway

Figure 9.8 AV re-entrant tachycardia (due to left posterior accessory AV pathway)

Table 9.1 The characteristics of atrioventricular re-entrant tachycardias

QRS complexes:
Regular
Rate 130–250 beats/min
Usually narrow
P waves:
Inverted, during or after each QRS complex

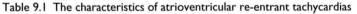

CLINICAL FEATURES

The arrhythmia is common. Attacks may start in infancy, childhood or adult life and often recur. The duration and frequency of attacks varies from patient to

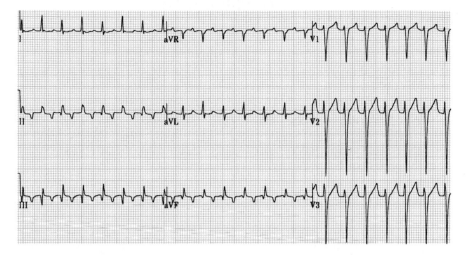

Figure 9.9 AV re-entrant tachycardia (due to posteroseptal accessory AV pathway)

patient. They may last for a few minutes or for many hours, and may occur several times per day or be separated by many months. In some patients, attacks are precipitated by exertion. In most, episodes can occur at rest or on exertion and can be brought on by trivial activities such as bending down.

TREATMENT

The patient should be reassured the tachycardia is not dangerous and that it is due to an electrical rather than structural cardiac abnormality; patients often fear the arrhythmia is due to coronary disease and that they are at risk from a heart attack.

Treatment is unnecessary for short episodes of tachycardia which do not cause distress.

Several treatments can be used to terminate or to prevent recurrence of the arrhythmia (Table 9.2).

Table 9.2 Summary of treatments for atrioventricular re-entrant tachycardias

Termination:
Vagal stimulation
Intravenous drugs, e g adenosine, verapamil
Cardioversion
Pacing (overdrive or programmed stimulation)
Prevention:
Drugs, e.g. sotalol, flecainide
Ablation of additional connection

VAGAL STIMULATION

The first approach to termination is vagal stimulation. An increase in vagal tone may temporarily slow conduction through the AV node and thereby interrupt the tachycardia circuit.

The Valsalva manoeuvre and carotid sinus massage are the best methods: they should be carried out with the patient lying down. The former is performed by the patient attempting to forcefully expire for 10–15 s while sealing the nose and mouth. Carotid massage is performed by firm digital pressure over one carotid artery at the level of the upper border of the thyroid cartilage for 5 s.

Eyeball pressure is widely quoted as a method for vagal stimulation but is very painful and should not be used.

INTRAVENOUS DRUGS

If vagal stimulation fails, the tachycardia can almost certainly be terminated by an intravenous injection of one of several drugs. Adenosine is the treatment of choice.

Adenosine

Adenosine is a potent blocker of AV nodal conduction which has an extremely short duration of action: 20 s. It is very effective in terminating AVNRT and AVRT (Figure 9.10).

It should be given as a rapid (2 s) intravenous bolus, followed by a saline flush. The initial dose in adults and in children is 3 mg and 0.05 mg/kg, respectively. If ineffective, further dosages of 6 mg (0.10 mg/kg) and, if necessary, 12 mg can be given after 1-min intervals up to a recommended maximum of 12 mg (0.25 mg/kg). Doses as high as 18 mg have been given without significant unwanted effect.

Many patients will experience chest tightness, dyspnoea and flushing, but the symptoms last less than 30 s. There may be complete AV block for a few seconds following termination of the tachycardia. A few ventricular ectopic beats may also occur. The drug does not have a negative inotropic action.

Adenosine can cause bronchospasm and avoidance is recommended in asthmatics.

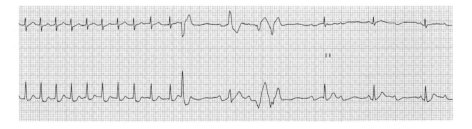

Figure 9.10 Following termination of AV nodal re-entrant tachycardia by adenosine, there are some ventricular ectopic beats and a short period of AV block

Verapamil

Intravenous verapamil (5–10 mg over 30 s) will usually restore sinus rhythm within a couple of minutes.

Verapamil must not be used if the patient has recently received an oral or intravenous beta-blocking drug (*see* Chapter 19).

OTHER DRUGS

Drugs such as sotalol, disopyramide and flecainide may also be effective (*see* Chapter 19).

ELECTRICAL METHODS

Pacing

Various pacing methods may terminate AV re-entrant tachycardias. The simplest is pacing the right atrium at a rate 20–30% faster than the tachycardia (overdrive pacing). On abrupt termination of pacing, sinus rhythm will often return; if unsuccessful, pacing should be repeated (Figure 9.11). There is a small risk of precipitating atrial fibrillation, which usually will not last for many minutes before sinus rhythm is restored. However, in patients with Wolff–Parkinson–White syndrome, atrial fibrillation might lead to a very fast ventricular response (see below).

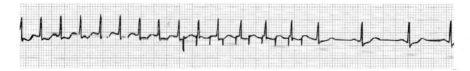

Figure 9.11 Termination of AV re-entrant tachycardia by rapid atrial pacing

More sophisticated methods require a programmable pacemaker, which allows the introduction of precisely timed extrastimuli (Figure 9.12). These methods can also be used on a long-term basis by implanting a pacemaker (Figure 9.13) but pacing has now been superceeded by radiofrequency ablation .

Cardioversion

If drugs are ineffective or if clinical circumstances necessitate an immediate return to sinus rhythm, cardioversion should be carried out (*see* chapter 20).

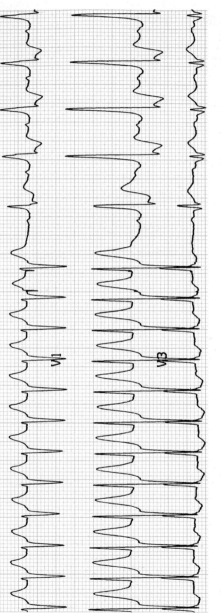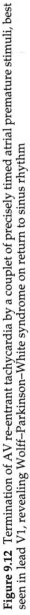

Figure 9.12 Termination of AV re-entrant tachycardia by a couplet of precisely timed atrial premature stimuli, best seen in lead V1, revealing Wolff–Parkinson–White syndrome on return to sinus rhythm

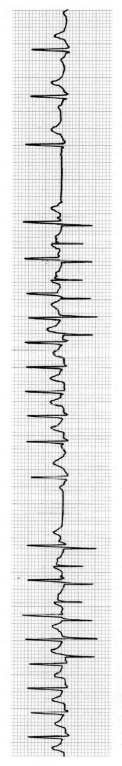

Figure 9.13 Implanted anti-tachycardia pacemaker. Automatic detection and termination of two episodes of AV re-entrant tachycardia

PREVENTION

There are two main approaches: drug therapy, or ablation of part of the re-entry circuit.

Drugs

Selection of a drug which is both effective and well tolerated is often a process of trial and error. Sotalol (160 mg daily) and flecainide (100 mg b.d.) are good first-line drugs. The patient should keep a record of the date and duration of any attacks so that the effect of therapy can be assessed.

Amiodarone is likely to be effective where other drugs have failed, but should be reserved for refractory cases where the need for tachycardia control outweighs the drug's possible unwanted effects.

Catheter ablation

Radiofrequency energy, delivered by a catheter introduced via a vein or artery, can be used to ablate an accessory pathway responsible for AVRT, or to modify the slow or fast AV nodal tract involved in AV nodal re-entrant tachycardia (*see* chapter 26). For many patients, this is the treatment of choice, offering a cure and obviating the need for anti-arrhythmic drugs. Success rates over 90% are being widely achieved and the risks are very low.

Main points

- AV re-entrant tachycardia requires the presence of a second connection between atria and ventricles in addition to the AV node.

- AVRT is due to an accessory AV pathway.

- AVNRT is caused by dual AV nodal pathways.

- Usually structural heart disease is absent.

- The ventricular rhythm is regular and QRS complexes usually narrow.

- Atrial activity, if seen, will be in the form of an inverted P wave after each QRS complex.

- Tachycardia can be terminated by vagal stimulation or adenosine.

- Radiofrequency ablation is now a first-line choice for the prevention of troublesome tachycardias.

Wolff–Parkinson–White syndrome

This syndrome is due to an accessory AV pathway, the same pathway, which, as discussed above, is the cause of an atrioventricular re-entrant tachycardia (AVRT). This connection is a strand of normal myocardium. It used to be called a bundle of Kent.

Normally the atria become electrically isolated from the ventricles during foetal development, apart from the AV junction (i.e. AV node plus bundle of His). Incomplete separation leads to an accessory AV pathway. The pathway may be situated anywhere across the groove between atria and ventricles. The most common site is the left free wall of the heart. Other locations are posteroseptal, right free wall and anteroseptal. In a minority of patients there is more than one accessory pathway.

Approximately 1.5–3 in each 1000 of the population have the electrocardiographic signs of Wolff–Parkinson–White syndrome, two-thirds of whom will experience cardiac arrhythmias. One survey reported 4 per 100 000 newly diagnosed cases per annum. The syndrome is more common in young people. With age, fibrosis may occasionally develop in the atrioventricular groove and block an accessory pathway.

To facilitate the common form of atrioventricular re-entrant tachycardia it is *only* necessary for the accessory pathway to conduct in a retrograde direction, i.e. from ventricles to atria. Many patients with AV re-entrant tachycardia have an accessory AV pathway which is only capable of ventriculoatrial conduction. In patients with the Wolff–Parkinson–White syndrome the pathway is *also* capable of anterograde conduction, i.e. from atria to ventricles. Unlike the AV node, the accessory connection does not delay conduction between atria and ventricles.

ECG CHARACTERISTICS

The characteristics of the Wolff–Parkinson–White syndrome are a short PR interval, a widened QRS complex due to the presence of a delta wave, and paroxysmal tachycardia (Figure 10.1).

During sinus rhythm, an atrial impulse will reach the ventricles via both the accessory pathway and the normal AV node. The AV node conducts relatively slowly. Therefore initial ventricular activation is solely due to accessory pathway conduction, which results in a shortened PR interval: ventricular pre-excitation. Because the accessory pathway is not connected to specialized conducting tissue (i.e. the His–Purkinje system), early ventricular activation will be slow, leading to slurring of the ventricular complex (i.e. a delta wave) rather than the brisk upstroke, which would result from rapid ventricular activation via the specialized conducting tissues. Once the atrial impulse has traversed the AV node, further ventricular activation will proceed normally. During sinus rhythm, therefore, the ventricular complex is a fusion between delta wave and normal QRS complex (Figure 10.1).

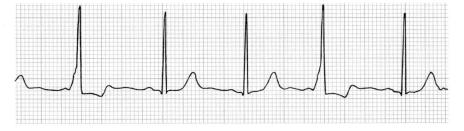

Figure 10.1 Wolff–Parkinson–White syndrome. In this patient, the accessory pathway conducts intermittently. The second, third and fifth complexes are normal, whereas the first and fourth complexes show the characteristic short PR interval and delta wave. By comparing pre-excited and normal beats, it can be seen how the delta wave both shortens the PR interval and broadens the ventricular complex

LOCATION OF ACCESSORY PATHWAY

The syndrome is classified into types A and B, depending on the ventricular complex in lead V1. If predominantly positive, it is type A and if negative, type B (Figures 10.2 and 10.3). Type A is caused by a left-sided accessory pathway.

Complex electrocardiographic algorithms have been devised for precise location of accessory pathways but none are completely reliable. A dominant delta wave in lead V1 indicates a left-sided pathway. A negative delta wave in leads III and aVF together with positive waves in leads V2 and V3 points to a posteroseptal pathway

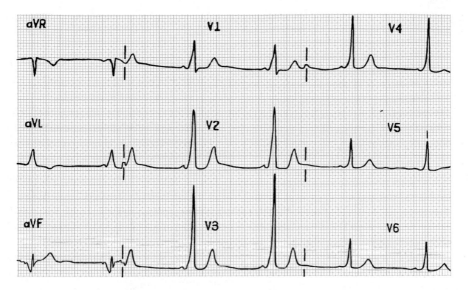

Figure 10.2 Type A Wolff–Parkinson–White syndrome. (The negative delta wave in lead aVF could be misinterpreted as a Q wave due to inferior myocardial infarction)

(*see* Figure 10.6b), while a right free wall pathway is usually associated with positive waves in leads II and III and a negative wave in lead V1.

ARRHYTHMIAS

Two main arrhythmias can occur in patients with the Wolff–Parkinson–White syndrome: atrial fibrillation and, more commonly, atrioventricular re-entrant tachycardia.

ATRIAL FIBRILLATION

In patients without pre-excitation the AV node protects the ventricles from the rapid atrial activity during atrial fibrillation (350–600 impulses/min). In the Wolff–Parkinson–White syndrome, the accessory pathway provides an additional route of access to the ventricles and can in some patients conduct very frequently. As a result, ventricular rates during atrial fibrillation are often very fast. Usually, most conducted impulses reach the ventricles via the accessory pathway and therefore lead to delta waves. The minority of impulses which reach the ventricles via the AV node produce normal QRS complexes. The resultant ECG will show the totally irregular ventricular response which is characteristic of atrial fibrillation. Some ventricular complexes will be normal; most will be delta waves (Figures 10.4 and 10.5).

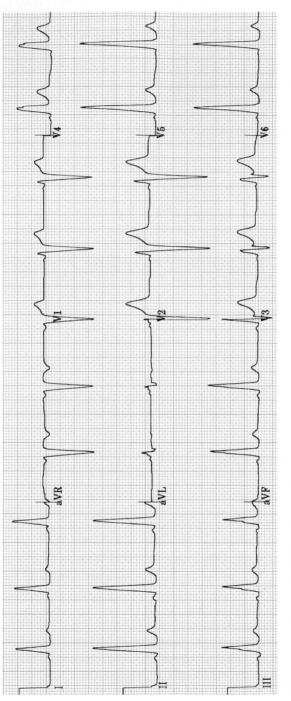
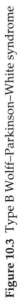

Figure 10.3 Type B Wolff–Parkinson–White syndrome

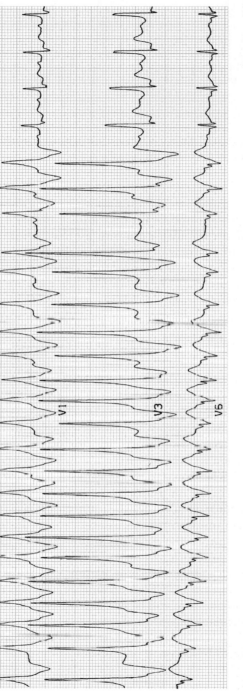
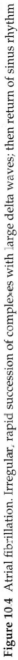

Figure 10.4 Atrial fibrillation. Irregular, rapid succession of complexes with large delta waves; then return of sinus rhythm

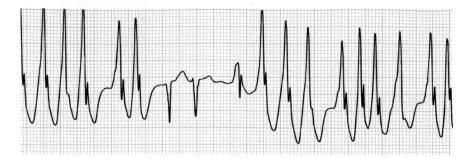

Figure 10.5 Atrial fibrillation. Most complexes are delta waves; the seventh and eighth complexes are narrow due to conduction via the AV node

A very rapid ventricular response to atrial fibrillation may cause heart failure or shock. If the ventricles are stimulated at a very fast rate, there is a risk of ventricular fibrillation. The risk of ventricular fibrillation is small and mainly affects those patients where the minimum interval between delta waves during atrial fibrillation is less than 250 ms (Figure 10.6). The risk is very low in asymptomatic patients and in those with intermittent accessory pathway conduction (Figure 10.1).

ATRIOVENTRICULAR RE-ENTRANT TACHYCARDIA

The AV node and accessory pathway differ in the time they take to recover after excitation. Usually, the AV node recovers first. If an atrial ectopic beat arises during sinus rhythm when the AV node has recovered but the accessory pathway is not yet capable of conduction, the resultant ventricular complex will clearly not have a delta wave and will be narrow. By the time the premature atrial impulse has traversed the AV junction and stimulated the ventricles, the accessory pathway will have recovered and will be able to conduct the impulse back to the atria. When the impulse reaches the atria, the AV junction will again be able to conduct and hence the impulse can repeatedly circulate between atria and ventricles, leading to an AV re-entrant tachycardia. Similarly, a ventricular ectopic beat during sinus rhythm can be conducted to the atria via the accessory pathway and thereby initiate AV re-entrant tachycardia.

The ECG during tachycardia will show narrow ventricular complexes (unless there is rate-related bundle branch block) in rapid regular succession (Figure 10.7).

Unlike atrial fibrillation, there will be no delta waves and, thus, there will be no clue from the ventricular complexes during tachycardia that the patient has Wolff–Parkinson–White syndrome. However, as discussed above, the timing of atrial activity during tachycardia, if identifiable, may point to the tachycardia mechanism. An accessory AV pathway is some distance from the AV junction. It therefore takes longer for an impulse to circulate and re-enter the atria. Hence the inverted P wave occurs roughly half way between QRS complexes (Figure 10.8). If inverted in lead I, the accessory pathway is likely to be left sided.

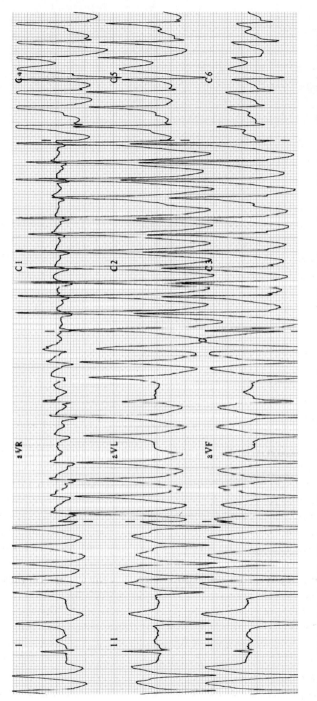

Figure 10.6 (a) Atrial fibrillation with a very rapid ventricular response. The minimum interval between delta waves is 200 ms. The totally irregular response excludes a diagnosis of ventricular tachycardia

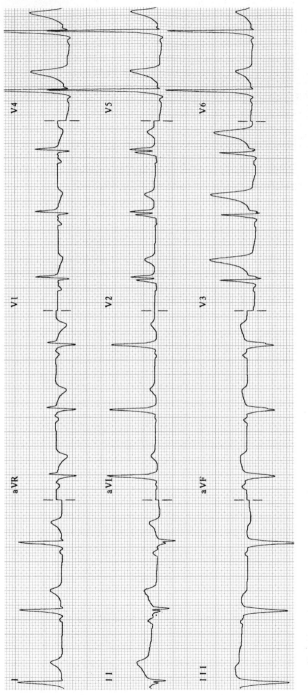

Figure 10.6 (b) The same patient in sinus rhythm. ECG suggests posteroseptal accessory pathway

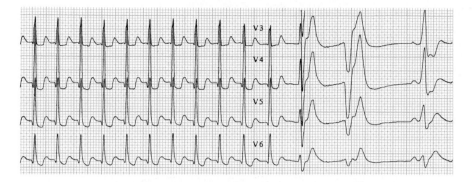

Figure 10.7 AV re-entrant tachycardia terminated by adenosine. After two ventricular ectopic beats, there is a sinus beat with short PR interval and delta wave

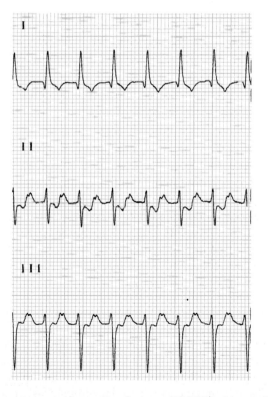

Figure 10.8 AV re-entrant tachycardia due to Wolff–Parkinson–White syndrome. Inverted P waves can be seen half way between QRS complexes. (The P wave is negative in lead I suggesting a left-sided pathway)

Antidromic tachycardia

Antidromic AV re-entrant tachycardia is much less common than the above-mentioned form of AV re-entrant tachycardia (which is termed orthodromic). The circulating impulse travels in the opposite direction: conduction from atria to ventricles is over the accessory AV pathway and return to the atria is via the AV node. Consequently, ventricular complexes will be in the form of large delta waves (Figure 10.9).

TREATMENT

Radiofrequency ablation of the accessory pathway (*see* chapter 26) should be considered in all symptomatic patients, particularly if drugs are ineffective or cannot be tolerated, or if there is a fast ventricular response to atrial fibrillation. Occasionally, ablation is indicated in asymptomatic patients by reason of their profession such as a pilot.

AV RE-ENTRANT TACHYCARDIA

Methods for the termination and prevention AV re-entrant tachycardia are appropriate whether or not the patient has pre-excitation during sinus rhythm (see above).

ATRIAL FIBRILLATION

During atrial fibrillation, most atrial impulses reach the ventricles via the accessory AV pathway. Thus AV nodal-blocking drugs such as digoxin and verapamil are of little use during atrial fibrillation in the Wolff–Parkinson–White syndrome. Indeed, both digoxin and verapamil can increase the frequency of conduction in the accessory pathway and therefore lead to a faster ventricular rate. These drugs should not be used in those patients who are capable of a rapid ventricular response in case a dangerously fast ventricular rate develops. In patients in whom atrial fibrillation has never occurred, and thus a fast response has not been excluded, the drugs should be avoided.

The simplest method of terminating atrial fibrillation is cardioversion, but this is not appropriate if the arrhythmia is frequently recurrent. If drugs are to be used, they must slow conduction in the accessory pathway, e.g. intravenous sotalol, flecainide, disopyramide or amiodarone. These drugs will slow the ventricular response to atrial fibrillation and will often restore sinus rhythm.

For prevention of atrial fibrillation, oral sotalol, flecainide, disopyramide or amiodarone are effective. In patients with a dangerously fast ventricular response to atrial fibrillation, the arrhythmia can be initiated by rapid atrial pacing once the patient is on anti-arrhythmic therapy to ensure the drug will slow the ventricular rate.

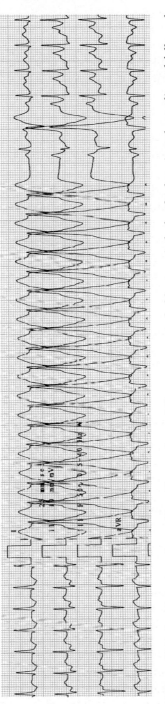

Figure 10.9 Antidromic tachycardia with very large delta waves, preceded by a period of orthodromic tachycardia and followed by sinus rhythm

Main points

- The Wolff–Parkinson–White syndrome is characterized by a short PR interval and a widened QRS complex owing to the presence of a delta wave. It is caused by an accessory AV pathway (bundle of Kent), which connects atrial and ventricular myocardium, bypassing the AV junction.

- Two main arrhythmias can occur: AV re-entrant tachycardia and atrial fibrillation.

- During atrioventricular re-entrant tachycardia, there will be no delta waves and thus no evidence from the ventricular complex of pre-excitation. Treatment is the same whether or not there is pre-excitation.

- During atrial fibrillation, most ventricular complexes are broad, owing to the presence of large delta waves. The ventricular rate is often very fast and there is a risk of ventricular fibrillation when the minimum interval between delta waves during atrial fibrillation is less than 250 ms. If the hallmark of atrial fibrillation (i.e. a totally irregular rhythm) is ignored, the arrhythmia may be mistaken for ventricular tachycardia.

- Since most atrial impulses are conducted to the ventricles via the accessory AV pathway during atrial fibrillation, AV nodal-blocking drugs (digoxin, verapamil) are not helpful and may be dangerous. Cardioversion is the simplest method for termination of atrial fibrillation. If a drug is used, it should slow conduction in the accessory pathway (e.g. sotalol, flecainide and amiodarone).

- Radiofrequency ablation should be considered in all symptomatic patients. Success rates are high and the risks low.

CHAPTER 11

Ventricular tachyarrhythmias

Ventricular tachycardia is defined as four or more ventricular ectopic beats in rapid succession (Figure 11.1). Ventricular tachycardias vary in rate, duration and frequency of recurrence. The consequences also vary. Some patients will develop shock or ventricular fibrillation whereas others may tolerate ventricular tachycardia with few or no symptoms.

There are two main types of ventricular tachycardia: monomorphic and polymorphic.

Monomorpic ventricular tachycardia (*see* chapter 12) is usually due to heart muscle damage but there are two specific tachycardias which occur in patients with structurally normal hearts.

Polymorphic ventricular tachycardia (*see* chapter 13) may also be caused by heart muscle damage. When associated with a prolonged QT interval, polymorphic ventricular tachycardia is termed 'torsade de pointes tachycardia'. There may be no structural heart disease. The arrhythmia results from abnormalities in ventricular repolarisation which can be aquired or inherited.

Ventricular fibrillation (*see* chapter 13) is usually a consequence of coronary or myocardial disease but occasionally is due to primary electrical disorders, including the recently described Brugada syndrome.

Difficulty is often encountered in distinguishing supraventricular from ventricular tachycardia. There are a number of pointers which can usually easily ascertain the origin of a tachycardia (*see* chapter 14).

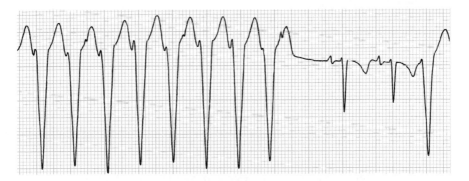

Figure 11.1 Ventricular tachycardia: a series of ventricular ectopic beats, followed by two sinus beats and a single ventricular ectopic beat

CHAPTER 12

Monomorphic ventricular tachycardia

ECG CHARACTERISTICS

The arrhythmia consists of a rapid succession of ventricular ectopic beats each with the same configuration, hence the term monomorphic (Figure 12.1). As with single ventricular ectopic beats, the complexes will be abnormal in shape, and the duration

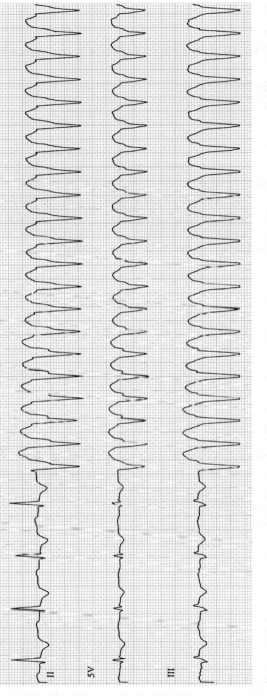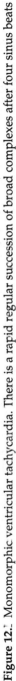

Figure 12. Monomorphic ventricular tachycardia. There is a rapid regular succession of broad complexes after four sinus beats

of each complex will be more than 0.12s and usually greater than 0.14s. The rhythm is regular unless there are capture beats (see below) which cause minor irregularities in the rhythm. The rate ranges from 120 to 250 beats/min.

ATRIAL ACTIVITY DURING VENTRICULAR TACHYCARDIA

With many ventricular tachycardias, the sinus node continues to initiate atrial activity which is therefore independent of, and slower than, ventricular activity (Figure 12.2). In others, the AV node conducts each ventricular impulse to the atria so a P wave follows the ventricular complex. The P wave is often concealed by the superimposed terminal portion of the ventricular complex (Figure 12.3). Rarely, second-degree block may occur at the AV junction so only some ventricular impulses are conducted to the atria.

Identification of independent atrial activity during tachycardia excludes an origin at AV node level or above, and will thus distinguish ventricular tachycardia from supraventricular tachycardia with broad ventricular complexes. There may be direct or indirect evidence of independent atrial activity.

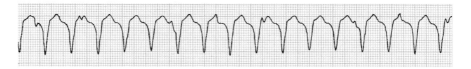

Figure 12.2 Ventricular tachycardia with direct evidence of independent atrial activity. P waves separated by intervals of 0.75 s can be seen after the 1st, 3rd, 6th, 8th, 10th, 13th, 15th and 17th ventricular complexes

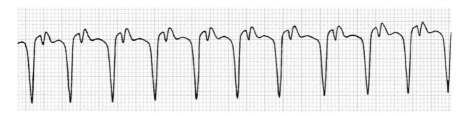

Figure 12.3 Ventricular tachycardia (lead aVF) with retrograde atrial activation. In this case, a P wave can be clearly seen to be superimposed on the T wave of each ventricular complex

Direct evidence of independent atrial activity

P waves at a slower rate than and dissociated from ventricular activity are direct evidence of independent atrial activity (Figure 12.2). Inevitably, some P waves will be concealed by superimposed ventricular complexes. Furthermore, not all leads will clearly show atrial activity. A rhythm strip is often inadequate and scrutiny of a simultaneous recording of several different leads may be necessary. Sometimes there will be doubt whether small waves on the ECG during tachycardia are caused by atrial activity. If they are, they will be separated by similar intervals, or multiples of that interval.

Indirect evidence of independent atrial activity

Capture or fusion beats are indirect evidence of atrial activity. Just one is sufficient to confirm ventricular tachycardia.

Capture beats occur when the timing of an atrial impulse during ventricular tachycardia is such that it can be transmitted via the AV junction and activate the ventricles before the next discharge from the ventricular focus. The resultant ventricular complex will be normal in shape and duration and will occur slightly earlier than the next ventricular ectopic beat would have been expected (Figure 12.10). Fusion beats are caused by a similar process. However, the atrial impulse activates the ventricles slightly later in the cardiac cycle leading to simultaneous activation of the ventricles by the transmitted atrial impulse and the ventricular focus. The result is a ventricular complex with an appearance intermediate between a normal QRS complex and a ventricular ectopic beat (Figure 12.4).

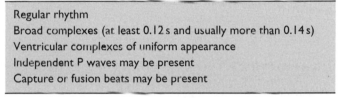

Table 12.1 Characteristics of monomorphic ventricular tachycardia

Regular rhythm
Broad complexes (at least 0.12 s and usually more than 0.14 s)
Ventricular complexes of uniform appearance
Independent P waves may be present
Capture or fusion beats may be present

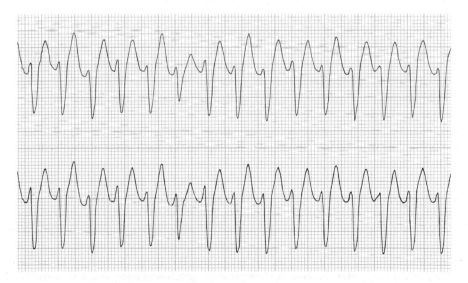

Figure 12.4 Ventricular tachycardia. The sixth complex is a fusion beat

CAUSES OF MONOMORPHIC VENTRICULAR TACHYCARDIA

Ventricular tachycardia is most often the result of myocardial damage from coronary heart disease or from cardiomyopathy. Below is a list of the main causes.

Table 12.2 Causes of ventricular tachycardia

Acute myocardial infarction or ischaemia
Past myocardial infarction
Dilated cardiomyopathy
Hypertrophic cardiomyopathy
Myocarditis
Arrhythmogenic right ventricular dysplasia
Mitral valve prolapse
Valvular heart disease
Repair of tetralogy of Fallot
Idiopathic

ARRHYTHMOGENIC RIGHT VENTRICULAR DYSPLASIA

Arrhythmogenic right ventricular dysplasia is caused by fatty and/or fibrous infiltration of the right ventricle. Sometimes only localized areas of the ventricle are affected. Impaired function can be demonstrated by angiography and sometimes by echocardiography. There is often some left ventricular impairment but less marked than right ventricular dysfunction. It is usually familial: the result of inheritance of an autosomal dominant gene. Males are more commonly affected. Because the tachycardia arises from the right ventricle, it has a left bundle branch block morphology (Figure 12.5a). Typically, during sinus rhythm there is T wave inversion in leads V1–V3 (Figure 12.5b).

Patients usually present between the ages of 20 and 50 years with palpitations, syncope or near syncope. Sudden death can occur and may be the first manifestation of this disorder.

ACCELERATED IDIOVENTRICULAR RHYTHM

Monomorphic ventricular tachycardia with a rate less than 120 beats/min is termed accelerated idioventricular rhythm or slow ventricular tachycardia (Figure 12.6). Acute myocardial infarction is the most common cause; treatment is unnecessary.

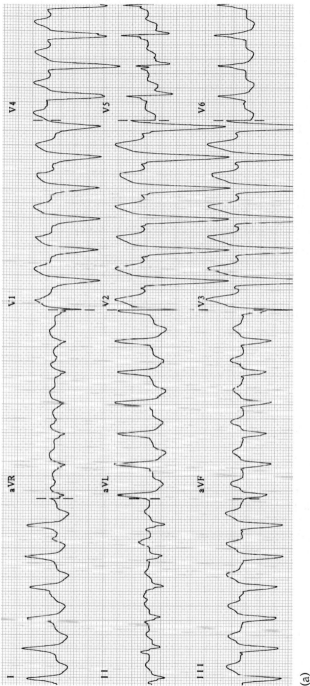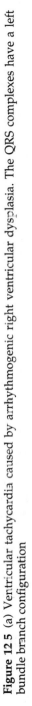

Figure 12.5 (a) Ventricular tachycardia caused by arrhythmogenic right ventricular dysplasia. The QRS complexes have a left bundle branch configuration

(a)

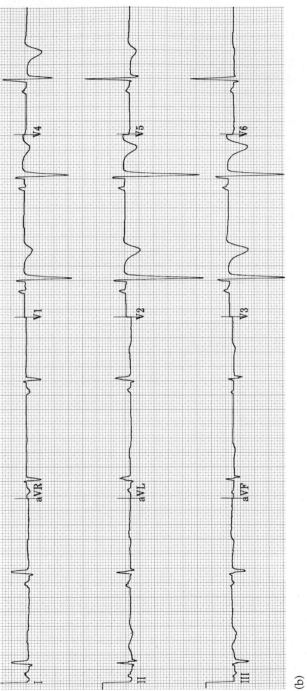

(b)

Figure 12.5 (b) The same patient with arrhythmogenic right ventricular dysplasia during sinus rhythm

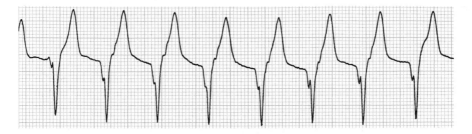

Figure 12.6 Accelerated idioventricular rhythm

NONSUSTAINED VENTRICULAR TACHYCARDIA

Nonsustained ventricular tachycardia is defined as three or more ventricular ectopic beats in succession at a rate in excess of 120 beats/min with return to normal rhythm within 30 s (Figure 12.7). It rarely causes symptoms but it is of prognostic significance in some groups of patients.

Many but not all studies have shown that patients with nonsustained ventricular tachycardia who have suffered a myocardial infarction and who have a left ventricular ejection fraction of less than 40% have a marked increased risk of death either from ventricular arrhythmia or heart failure. In dilated cardiomyopathy, there is a slight increase in risk of sudden death in those with nonsustained ventricular tachycardia. The arrhythmia is associated with a significant increased risk in symptomatic patients with hypertrophic cardiomyopathy. Nonsustained ventricular tachycardia rarely occurs in subjects without structural heart disease and is not associated with risk.

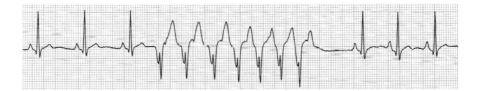

Figure 12.7 Nonsustained ventricular tachycardia

VENTRICULAR TACHYCARDIAS NOT DUE TO STRUCTURAL HEART DISEASE

There are two important ventricular tachycardias which can arise in structurally normal hearts. The more common one arises from the right ventricle and the other from the left ventricle. Recognition is important because they are associated with a good prognosis, their typical configurations point strongly to the heart being structurally normal, and because they are easily amenable to radiofrequency ablation if required for symptomatic purposes (*see* chapter 26).

RIGHT VENTRICULAR OUTFLOW TRACT TACHYCARDIA

This tachycardia has a characteristic ECG appearance which reflects its origin in the right ventricular outflow tract, just below the pulmonary valve. Because it arises in the right ventricle the complexes are similar to those seen during left bundle branch block and, because the impulse spreads inferiorly from beneath the pulmonary valve, there is an inferior frontal QRS axis, i.e. right axis deviation (Figure 12.8).

There are two types of clinical presentation. Either the tachycardia is paroxysmal and is provoked by effort, or it occurs at rest and is repetitive and nonsustained. In contrast to most ventricular tachycardias, it may be terminated by adenosine and verapamil.

In some patients, frequent ectopic beats rather than tachycardia arise from the right ventriclular outflow tract (Figure 12.9).

Rarely, a similar tachycardia arises from the left ventricular outflow tract. In contrast to right ventricular outflow tract tachycardia, leads V1–V3 are usually positive.

FASCICULAR TACHYCARDIA

Fascicular tachycardia is an uncommon arrhythmia which arises from the posterior fascicle or, more rarely, from the anterior fascicle of the left bundle branch.

A posterior fascicular origin results in ventricular complexes during tachycardia with a right bundle branch block and left axis configuration (Figure 12.10), while an anterior fascicular origin leads to right bundle branch block with right axis deviation. Because the origin is within the specialized conducting system, the ventricular complexes are of relatively short duration (0.12 s), sometimes leading to confusion with supraventricular tachycardia. The right bundle branch configuration may be atypical, for example, there is a small q wave rather than a primary r wave.

Like right ventricular outflow tract tachycardia, it can be terminated by verapamil (but not adenosine).

MECHANISMS OF VENTRICULAR TACHYCARDIAS

Two main mechanisms cause tachycardias. One is re-entry: this is the commonest mechanism for ventricular tachycardia. The other is enhanced automaticity which may be spontaneous or triggered.

RE-ENTRY

Two conditions are necessary for a re-entrant tachycardia to occur. The first is the presence of a potential circuit made up of two pathways of tissue with differing

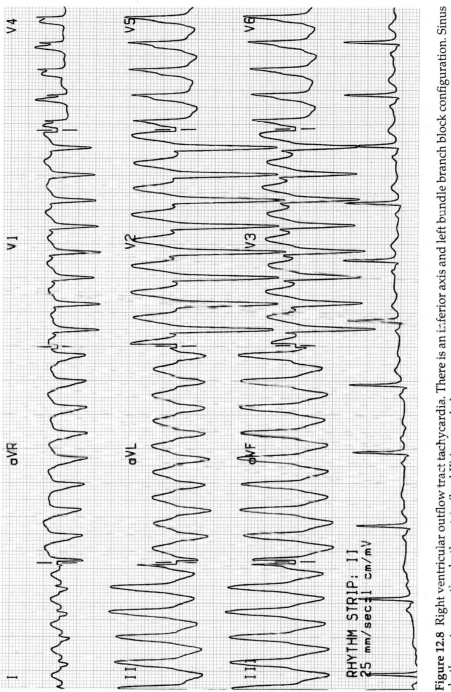

Figure 12.8 Right ventricular outflow tract tachycardia. There is an inferior axis and left bundle branch block configuration. Sinus rhythm returns as the rhythm strip (lead II) is recorded.

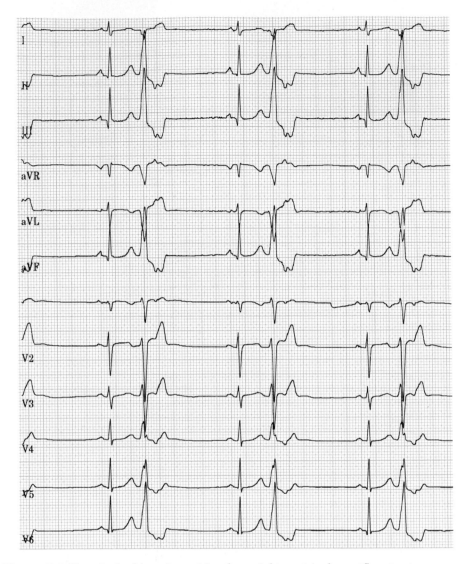

Figure 12.9 Ventricular bigeminy arising from right ventricular outflow tract

electrical characteristics. The second is transient or permanent block in one direction in one of the pathways, so an impulse can be conducted along one pathway and return in the opposite direction via the other pathway, thereby re-entering the circuit. The activating impulse is repeatedly conducted around the circuit, exciting the surrounding myocardium at a rapid rate.

In ventricular tachycardia, fibrosis or ischaemia may cause delay in activation and hence recovery of an area of myocardium. Tachycardia results when a premature beat arrives at the abnormal area to find it is refractory to excitation following the last heart beat. The impulse is conducted around the damaged area by

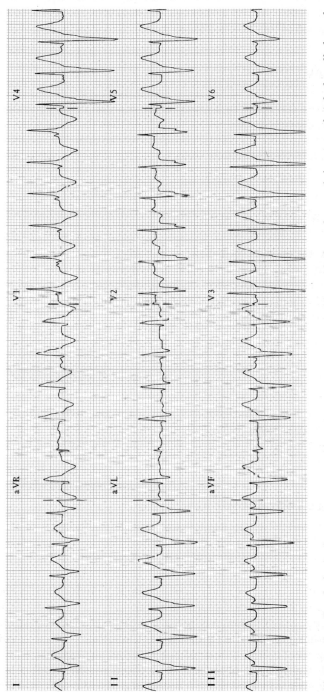

Figure 12.10 Fascicular tachycardia arising from the posterior fascicle. The complexes have a left axis and right bundle branch block configuration. The eighth complex is a capture beat

the adjacent normally responsive myocardium. By the time the impulse has circumvented the damaged area, the abnormal myocardium has become excitable again and conducts the impulse in the opposite direction giving rise to a re-entrant circuit. Perpetuation of this process results in ventricular tachycardia.

ENHANCED AUTOMATICITY

Damage or disease can result in a group of myocardial cells acquiring enhanced automaticity, i.e. the cells discharge at a higher rate than the sinus node, taking over control of the heart rhythm. Enhanced automaticity can either be spontaneous or be triggered by after-depolarizations which lead to early reactivation of the myocardium.

INITIATION OF TACHYCARDIA

A re-entrant circuit or focus of enhanced automaticity provide the substrate for ventricular tachycardia. Initiation of the arrhythmia is usually triggered by an ectopic beat. Ischaemia, increased sympathetic nervous system activity or electrolyte imbalance may influence the arrhythmia substrate and may account for a tachycardia occurring at a particular time.

INVESTIGATIONS

The nature and extent of investigations has to be tailored to the individual clinical situation. The aims should be to identify the cause, which may well be of therapeutic or prognostic importance, and to assess the role and efficacy of any therapy that may be indicated.

12-LEAD ELECTROCARDIOGRAM

Whenever possible, a 12-lead electrocardiogram during tachycardia should be recorded and saved. It may point to the origin of the tachycardia. Furthermore, if electrophysiological studies are to be carried out, it is important to know that a tachycardia induced during the study has the same morphology and is therefore the same arrhythmia as has occurred spontaneously.

An ECG during sinus rhythm may reveal the cause of tachycardia, e.g. demonstrating myocardial infarction or a prolonged QT interval.

The configuration of the ventricular complex during tachycardia gives a clue as to its site of origin. A positive complex in lead V1 points to a left ventricular source. If complexes are negative in V4–V6, a left ventricular apical origin is likely, while Q waves in the inferior leads suggest that the tachycardia is arising from the base of the left ventricle.

IMAGING

Echocardiography may help establish the cause of the arrhythmia. For example, by demonstrating dilated or hypertrophic cardiomyopathy, or right ventricular dysplasia.

Coronary angiography is often indicated, particularly if myocardial ischaemia might be the cause of the arrhythmia or if surgery is contemplated.

AMBULATORY ELECTROCARDIOGRAPHY

Ambulatory electrocardiography will help assess the frequency and duration of episodes of ventricular tachycardia and the effect of therapy in those patients who have had frequent episodes.

Occasionally, ventricular tachycardia is triggered by bradycardia. This may be revealed by ambulatory electrocardiography. Prevention of bradycardia will often prevent ventricular tachycardia.

EXERCISE TESTING

Exercise-induced tachycardia is common. An exercise test can be useful in its diagnosis and response to therapy.

Most anti-arrhythmic drugs can in some patients be pro-arrhythmic (see chapter 19). A pro-arrhythmic effect may only be apparent during exercise. As a rule, patients who receive long-term therapy to prevent ventricular tachycardia should undergo exercise testing.

ELECTROPHYSIOLOGICAL STUDY

Stimulation of the ventricles with up to three precisely timed premature stimuli delivered by a pacing lead, usually introduced via the femoral vein, will often induce ventricular tachycardia in patients who are prone to this arrhythmia. Drug therapy which then prevents reinduction of the arrhythmia or at least increases the cycle length during tachycardia by over 100 ms has been shown to have a favourable effect on prognosis. However, serial testing may be necessary to identify an effective drug, and not infrequently all anti-arrhythmic drugs will be found to be ineffective.

There are reservations about the predictive value of electrophysiological testing. The more aggressive the stimulation protocol in terms of the number of stimuli and the rate of stimulation, the easier it is to induce a ventricular arrhythmia. It is not clear which stimulation protocol has the best predictive accuracy. The results of a ventricular stimulation study are not always reproducible. There is doubt about the significance of induction of nonsustained ventricular tachycardia. Furthermore, it does not necessarily follow that the oral preparation of a drug that has proved effective when given intravenously during an electrophysiological test will prevent spontaneous ventricular arrhythmias. Amiodarone may prevent spontaneous ventricular tachycardia and yet the arrhythmia may still be inducible, though usually at a relatively slow rate, at electrophysiological testing.

SIGNAL-AVERAGED ELECTROCARDIOGRAPHY

Late potentials are low-voltage, high-frequency signals in the terminal portion of the QRS complex. They indicate an area of delayed myocardial activation and are commonly found in patients subject to ventricular tachycardia caused by a re-entrant mechanism. They are demonstrated by signal-averaged electrocardiography. The ECG is recorded with an orthogonal system: leads are placed in the fourth intercostal space in both midaxillary lines, on the front (lead V2 position) and back of chest, and top and bottom of the sternum. Computerized signal averaging and appropriate filtering of a series of QRS complexes eliminate electrical noise, which is random, and the main part of the QRS complex and thereby demonstrate late potentials (Figure 12.11).

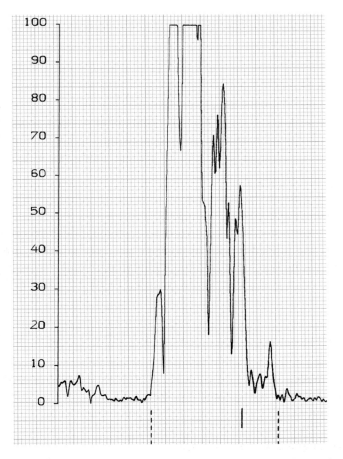

Figure 12.11 Signal-averaged electrocardiogram. Shaded area indicates late potential. Filtered QRS = 167 ms, root mean square of terminal 40 ms = 7 microvolt and duration of high-frequency low-amplitude signals in terminal 40 ms = 48 ms

Widely used criteria for late potentials are the presence of two of the following three observations:

1. filtered QRS duration > 110 ms;
2. root mean square of last 40 ms of QRS complex <25 ms;
3. duration of terminal portion of QRS complex <40 microvolts exceeds 32 ms.

Late potentials indicate the presence of the substrate for ventricular tachycardia, i.e. an area of slowed conduction, not that spontaneous ventricular tachycardia will necessarily occur. In patients who present with ventricular tachycardia, late potentials show the arrhythmia should be inducible at electrophysiological study. Late potentials after myocardial infarction point to a poor prognosis, particularly where there is evidence of extensive myocardial damage.

Rarely, a late potential may be apparent on routine electrocardiography, termed an epsilon wave (Figure 12.12).

PROGNOSIS

Ventricular tachycardia that is not due to an acute event such as acute myocardial infarction or drug toxicity is very likely to recur.

The prognosis of ventricular tachycardia depends on the cause and the resultant symptoms and haemodynamic disturbance. Idiopathic tachycardias such as right ventricular outflow tract and fascicular tachycardias are associated with low risk, while tachycardias caused by myocardial infarction or cardio-myopathy, whether dilated or hypertrophic, have a poor prognosis. Many studies have shown that one of the best predictors of prognosis is the degree of left ventricular impairment. Patients with an ejection fraction of less than 35% have a poor prognosis.

Ventricular tachycardias that cause cardiac arrest, syncope or severe hypotension have a worse prognosis than tachycardias which merely cause palpitation, and which are usually less fast.

TREATMENT

Choice of treatment depends on what symptoms the arrhythmia causes, whether the arrhythmia is likely to recur and the prognosis.

TERMINATION OF TACHYCARDIA

Options include cardioversion, drugs and pacing.

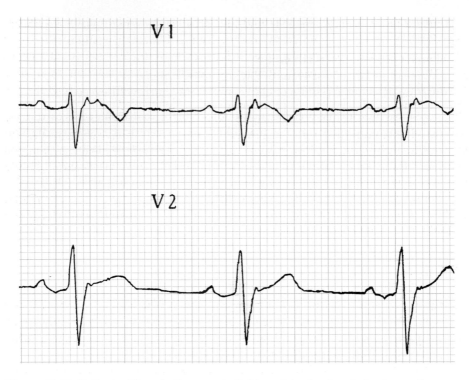

Figure 12.12 Patient with arrhythmogenic right ventricular dysplasia. An epsilon wave can be seen in the terminal portion of the QRS complex in lead V1

Cardioversion

If sustained ventricular tachycardia causes cardiac arrest or shock, immediate cardioversion is necessary (*see* chapter 20). Cardioversion should also be undertaken if anti-arrhythmic drugs are ineffective, contraindicated or cause haemodynamic deterioration without restoring normal rhythm.

Anti-arrhythmic drugs

Lignocaine is the first-line drug to stop ventricular tachycardia. Other drugs that are commonly used are sotalol, disopyramide and flecainide. These are markedly negatively inotropic (i.e. they can reduce the force of myocardial contraction) and are best avoided in patients with heart failure or in those known to have extensive myocardial damage. In general, no more than two drugs should be given before considering alternative methods of arrhythmia termination.

Amiodarone is a very useful second-line drug. It does not have a significant negative inotropic action and is extremely effective. However, it seldom works 'at the end of a needle' and can take up to 24 h to act. If ventricular tachycardia keeps recurring, it may be worth using amiodarone despite its delayed action rather than risking the complications associated with other less effective drugs, even if cardioversion or pacing is required while amiodarone is taking effect.

Though verapamil is effective in controlling supraventricular tachycardia, it is, except for fascicular and right ventricular outflow tract tachycardia, useless in ventricular tachycardia and may cause severe hypotension. It cannot be emphasized too strongly that it is dangerous practice to use the drug as a therapeutic test to ascertain the origin of a tachycardia with broad QRS complexes.

In contrast to most ventricular tachycardias, both fascicular and right ventricular outflow tract tachycardia may be terminated by verapamil and the latter arrhythmia may also respond to adenosine.

Pacing

Pacing can sometimes be successful in terminating ventricular tachycardia (Figure 12.13). It should be considered when drugs are ineffective, when frequently recurrent tachycardia necessitates multiple cardioversions or when a temporary pacing wire is already in place for treatment of a bradycardia.

The usual method is overdrive right ventricular pacing. A burst for a few seconds at a rate 10–30% in excess of that of the tachycardia will often terminate the arrhythmia. However, there is a significant risk of accelerating the tachycardia or precipitating ventricular fibrillation, in which case immediate cardioversion will be necessary.

In some patients, where there is a high risk should ventricular tachycardia recur or anti-arrhythmic drugs are ineffective, an automatic implantable cardiovertor defibrillator may be indicated (see chapter 25).

PREVENTION OF RECURRENCE OF VENTRICULAR TACHYCARDIA

Intravenous drugs

Blood levels of most anti-arrhythmic drugs fall rapidly after a single bolus. After a bolus has restored sinus rhythm it is usual to give a continuous infusion of the drug. This makes sense if ventricular tachycardia is expected to recur within a short period, e.g. after acute myocardial infarction. However, it is pointless to set up an infusion if either the bolus has failed or if the tachycardia is known to occur infrequently.

Oral drugs

Unless ventricular tachycardia occurs during acute myocardial infarction or other acute events, recurrence is likely and long-term therapy is indicated. Therapy is

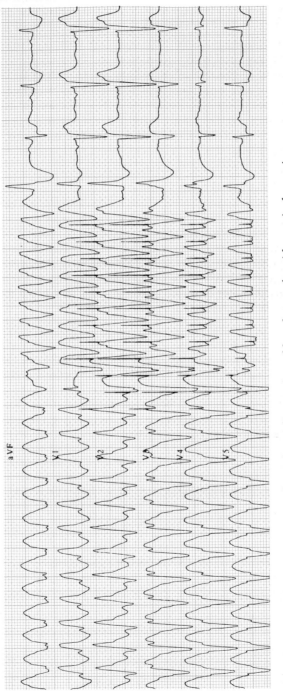

Figure 12.13 Monomorphic ventricular tachycardia terminated by a burst of rapid ventricular pacing

particularly important if the arrhythmia is associated with significant structural heart disease or has caused marked hypotension or shock, since the prognosis without treatment is poor.

Several drugs may be useful: sotalol, disopyramide, flecainide and amiodarone. When ventricular tachycardia has occurred on exertion, beta-blockers should be tried first.

Disopyramide, flecainide and beta-blockers may precipitate heart failure in patients with extensive myocardial damage. Amiodarone is by far the most effective drug and can be given to patients with poor ventricular function but it can cause a number of unwanted effects. In patients who are at high risk from further arrhythmias it would seem reasonable to use amiodarone and consider alternatives if major side-effects occur.

Ambulatory electrocardiography has been compared with programmed electrical stimulation in patients presenting with ventricular tachycardia who had 10 or more ventricular extrasystoles per hour to see which method could best predict anti-arrhythmic efficacy. Suppression of extrasystoles was found to be as predictive of anti-arrhythmic efficacy as prevention of inducibility of ventricular tachycardia by programmed electrical stimulation. However, neither method was found to be very reliable. Notably, sotalol was found to be a more effective anti-arrhythmic drug than mexiletine, pirmenolol, procainamide and propafenone.

The author's 'first-line' drugs to prevent ventricular tachycardia are sotalol and amiodarone.

Pacing

Sometimes ventricular tachycardia arises during bradycardia. If the heart rate is low, e.g. less than 50 beats/min, the rate should be increased by pacing before drugs are given; often pacing alone will prevent ventricular tachycardia. Pacing at a rate of 80–90 beats/min together with drugs may prevent ventricular tachycardia when the rate during sinus rhythm is relatively slow, e.g. 50–70 beats/min.

Catheter ablation

Delivery of radiofrequency energy via a catheter electrode to the site of origin of tachycardia is very effective in right ventricular outflow tract and fascicular tachycardias. It should be considered when troublesome symptoms occur, particularly since oral anti-arrhythmic drugs are rarely effective.

Modest rates of success have been achieved with some other ventricular tachycardias such as arrhythmogenic right ventricular dysplasia and in incessant tachycardia caused by myocardial infarction.

Surgery

There are several surgical techniques which involve the excision or isolation of the arrhythmia focus. However, potential candidates for surgery often have impaired myocardial function. Cardiopulmonary bypass surgery carries a substantial risk when myocardial function is poor since ventriculotomy may worsen function. Only a few cardiac centres routinely perform surgery for ventricular tachycardia.

There are reports that myocardial revascularization alone may reduce the incidence of ventricular arrhythmias in some patients with coronary heart disease.

Occasionally, life-threatening, resistant ventricular arrhythmias are an indication for cardiac transplantation.

ASSESSMENT OF EFFICACY

Whatever treatment is chosen, it is important to ensure it is effective in preventing a recurrence of ventricular tachycardia. If the tachycardia has been frequent, then monitoring the ECG at the bedside or using ambulatory electrocardiography is the best method of assessing efficacy. If ventricular tachycardia has been infrequent, then it is unlikely that ECG monitoring will reflect anti-arrhythmic control. Exercise ECG testing and electrophysiological testing should be considered.

Most anti-arrhythmic drugs can be pro-arrhythmic. Class IC drugs (*see* chapter 19) are the main culprits and patients with extensive myocardial damage the most susceptible. If no progress is being made in maintaining normal rhythm or there are new arrhythmias, a pro-arrhythmic effect should be considered.

Main points

- Monomorphic ventricular tachycardia consists of a rapid, regular succession of ventricular extrasystoles each with the same configuration. The duration exceeds 0.12 s and is usually greater than 0.14 s.

- The presence of P waves dissociated from ventricular activity or of fusion or capture beats indicates independent atrial activity and confirms ventricular tachycardia.

- The common causes of ventricular tachycardia are myocardial damage from coronary artery disease or from cardiomyopathy.

- Right ventricular outflow tract and fascicular tachycardia arise in patients with structurally normal hearts and are amenable to radiofrequency ablation.

- If the tachycardia causes shock, prompt cardioversion is indicated.

- Lignocaine is the first-line drug for intravenous use. Generally, no more than two drugs should be tried before resorting to amiodarone or nonpharmacological methods of treatment. Verapamil should not be given except for right ventricular outflow tract and fascicular tachycardias.

- It is important to try to ensure that long-term anti-arrhythmic therapy is effective since ventricular tachycardia is often a recurrent problem and may lead to sudden death.

- Accelerated idioventricular rhythm is ventricular tachycardia at a rate less than 120 beats/min. Treatment is not required.

- Wherever possible, obtain and save a 12-lead ECG during tachycardia.

CHAPTER 13

Polymorphic tachycardia and ventricular fibrillation

POLYMORPHIC TACHYCARDIA

Whereas monomorphic ventricular tachycardia consists of a rapid succession of ventricular ectopic beats each with the same configuration, polymorphic tachycardia is characterized by repeated progressive changes in the QRS complex so the complexes 'twist' about the baseline (Figure 13.1). It may result from acute myocardial infarction and from other causes of myocardial damage (Figure 13.2). In these situations the QT interval during sinus rhythm is normal and the management of the arrhythmia is the same as for monomorphic ventricular tachycardia.

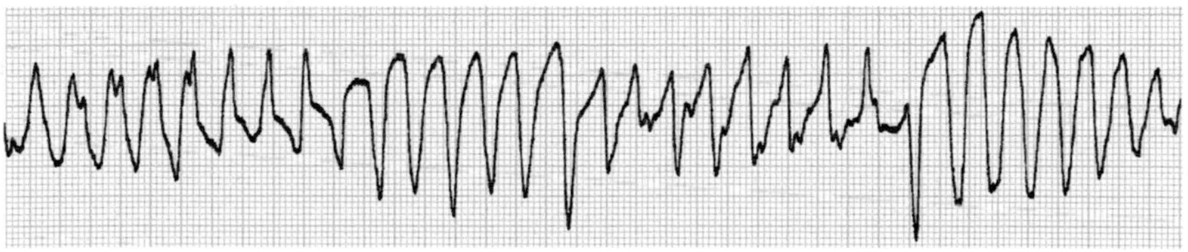

Figure 13.1 Polymorphic ventricular tachycardia

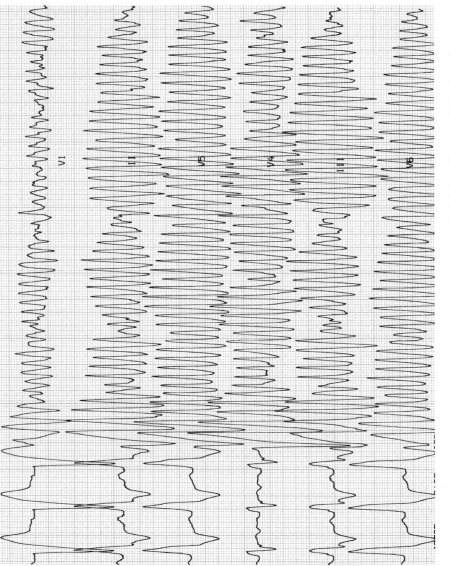
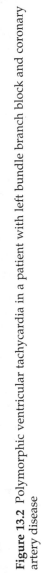

Figure 13.2 Polymorphic ventricular tachycardia in a patient with left bundle branch block and coronary artery disease

TORSADE DE POINTES TACHYCARDIA

This term refers to polymorphic ventricular tachycardia when the QT interval is prolonged in between episodes of the arrhythmia (Figure 13.3). Often there are prominent U waves. Recognition is important because anti-arrhythmic drugs may aggravate the tachycardia and because correction of its cause should prevent it.

The arrhythmia is caused by bradycardia, or by drugs or disorders that lead to abnormal ventricular repolarisation (Table 13.1). Usually it is nonsustained and repetitive but can deteriorate to ventricular fibrillation. Onset usually follows a pause in rhythm caused by bradycardia or following an ectopic beat.

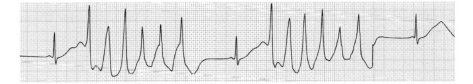

Figure 13.3 Two episodes of torsade de pointes tachycardia during sinus bradycardia: there is marked QT prolongation

Table 13.1 Causes of torsade de pointes tachycardia

Bradycardia due to sick sinus syndrome or atrioventricular block
Congenital prolongation of the QT interval
Hypokalaemia, hypomagnesaemia
Anti-arrhythmic drugs, e.g. quinidine, disopyramide, sotalol, amiodarone, ibutilide, dofetilide
Non-anti-arrhythmic drugs, e.g. prenylamine, bepridil, cisapride, tricyclic antidepressants, erythromycin, thioridazine, terfenadine, probucol
Anorexia nervosa

QT INTERVAL

The QT interval is a measure of the duration of ventricular repolarization. It is measured from the onset of the QRS complex to the end of the T wave. Precise measurement is difficult because the timing of these events varies from ECG lead to lead and because it can be difficult to define the point at which the T wave ends and U wave starts (Figure 13.4).

Prolongation of the QT interval may be due to either uniform prolongation of the process of repolarization throughout the myocardium, or variation in the rates of repolarization in disparate regions of myocardium. The latter situation is the one likely to cause ventricular arrhythmias.

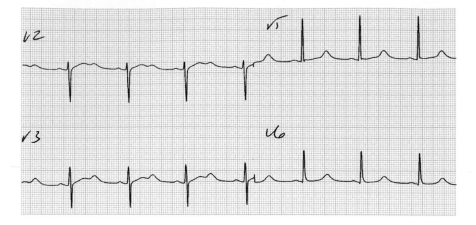

Figure 13.4 Apparent QT prolongation seen in leads V5 and V6 due to large U waves best seen in lead V3

The QT interval normally shortens with increasing heart rate, partly due to the increase in rate itself and partly due to the increase in sympathetic nervous system activity associated with sinus tachycardia. When measuring the QT interval it is necessary to correct the measured interval for heart rate. The corrected QT interval (QTc) is usually calculated by dividing the square root of the cycle length into the measured QT interval. The normal QTc does not exceed 0.44 s (Figure 13.5).

During exercise in patients with congenital QT prolongation, the QT interval may not shorten, and may prolong.

MANAGEMENT

Treatment consists of reversal of the cause where possible, and cardiac pacing. Intravenous magnesium sulphate may be effective, even when serum magnesium is normal (8 mmol stat; 2.5 mmol/h infusion).

Anti-arrhythmic drugs should be stopped. Increasing the heart rate to 100 beats/min by pacing will often prevent the tachycardia while the drug(s) are being excreted or metabolized.

CONGENITAL PROLONGATION OF THE QT INTERVAL

The Romano–Ward syndrome and the Jervell and Lange-Nielson syndrome are two conditions in which there is congenital prolongation of the QT interval and a tendency to ventricular tachycardia, usually polymorphic. The former is caused by a dominant gene; the latter is due to a recessive gene and is associated with nerve deafness. In addition, a similar but nonfamilial syndrome does occur sporadically.

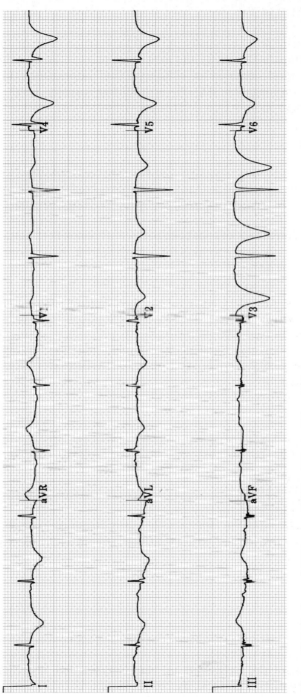

Figure 13.5 Prolonged QT interval. QT = 506 ms; QTc = 538 ms

It is now appreciated that the congenital long QT syndromes are caused by genetic abnormalities which control the functions of cardiac potassium and sodium ion channels. At least five genes have been identified and each gene has been associated with a number of different mutations.

Ventricular tachycardia is usually induced by exertion or emotion as a result of high levels of sympathetic activity and may cause syncope. Sudden death can occur. Symptoms are most common in childhood and adolescence. In one type of congenital QT prolongation (LQT2), arrhythmias usually result from sudden auditory stimuli. In another type (LQT3), arrhythmias occur during sleep.

Treatment

Full beta-blockade is often effective. Cardiac pacing in addition to beta-blockers should be considered in those patients with marked bradycardia prior to or because of beta-blockers. Asymptomatic patients who are young should receive a beta-blocker.

Left cervical sympathectomy has been performed where beta-blockade has failed. Occasionally, it is necessary to implant a cardiovertor defibrillator, especially in survivors of cardiac arrest.

Patients should be advised to avoid, if possible, drugs which may enhance sympathetic nervous system activity such as decongestants, midodrine, medications for asthma and fenfluramine. Drugs listed in Table 13.1 should also be considered.

It has been suggested that patients who develop torsade de pointes tachycardia as a result of a drug may have the same genetic abnormalities of cardiac ion channels that cause the congenital long QT syndromes but in a subclinical form. Females are more susceptible.

VENTRICULAR FIBRILLATION

ECG CHARACTERISTICS

Ventricular fibrillation is the rapid, totally incoordinate contraction of ventricular myocardial fibres. This is reflected in the ECG by irregular, chaotic electrical activity (Figure 13.6).

Ventricular fibrillation causes circulatory arrest. Unconsciousness develops within 10–20 s.

CAUSES

Ninety per cent of deaths caused by acute myocardial infarction are due to ventricular fibrillation. The incidence of fibrillation is highest in the first hour. Ventricular fibrillation can also occur late after infarction and, in patients with severe coronary artery disease, without myocardial infarction; it may be the first

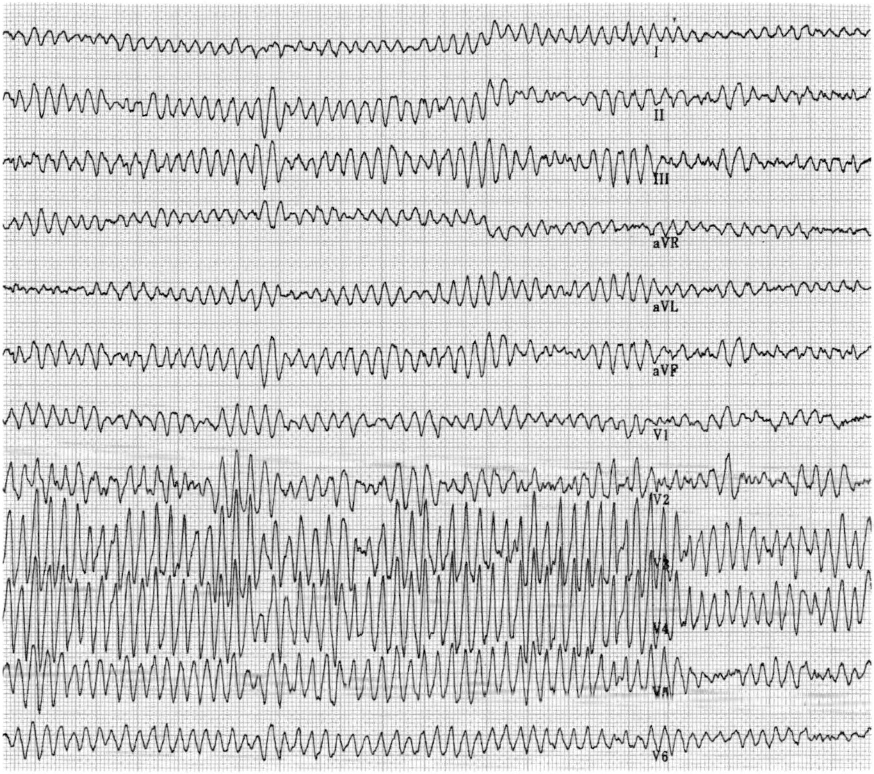

Figure 13.6 Ventricular fibrillation. Unusually, a full 12-lead ECG was obtained during ventricular fibrillation

clinical manifestation of the disease. The arrhythmia can result from many other cardiac disorders such as myocarditis and the cardiomyopathies. It may result from a primary electrical disorder (see Brugada syndrome, below).

It is usually initiated by a ventricular ectopic beat but can arise during a pause in cardiac rhythm or result from monomorphic or polymorphic ventricular tachycardia.

PRIMARY AND SECONDARY VENTRICULAR FIBRILLATION

If ventricular fibrillation develops in a heart that was functioning satisfactorily during normal rhythm it is termed 'primary' fibrillation, whereas if it occurs in the context of cardiac failure or cardiogenic shock, it is termed 'secondary'. Successful defibrillation is less likely in secondary ventricular fibrillation.

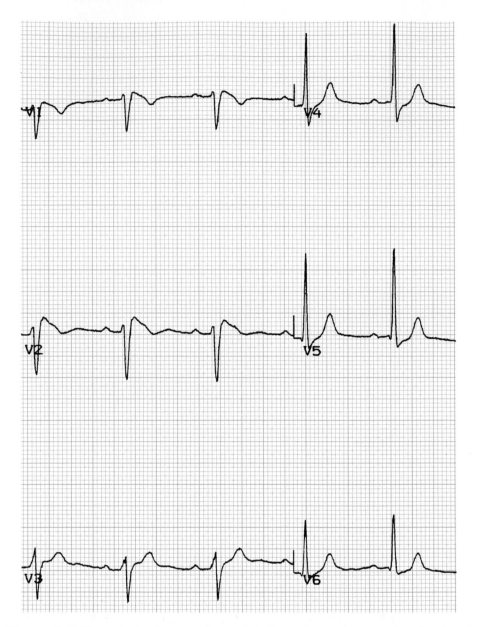

Figure 13.7 Chest leads from patient with Brugada syndrome who developed ventricular fibrillation while driving

TREATMENT

Rarely ventricular fibrillation is a brief event, spontaneously reverting to normal rhythm. Otherwise, without prompt treatment, irreversible cerebral and myocardial damage will quickly ensue.

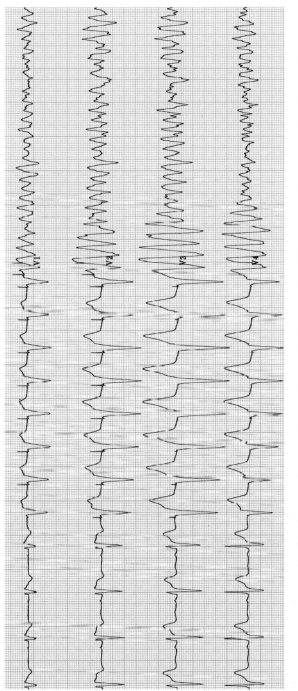

Figure 13.8 Asymptomatic patient with Brugada syndrome (leads V1–V4) who developed ventricular fibrillation during a ventricular stimulation study: after eight paced beats at 120 beats/min, a couplet of premature stimuli initiated ventricular fibrillation.

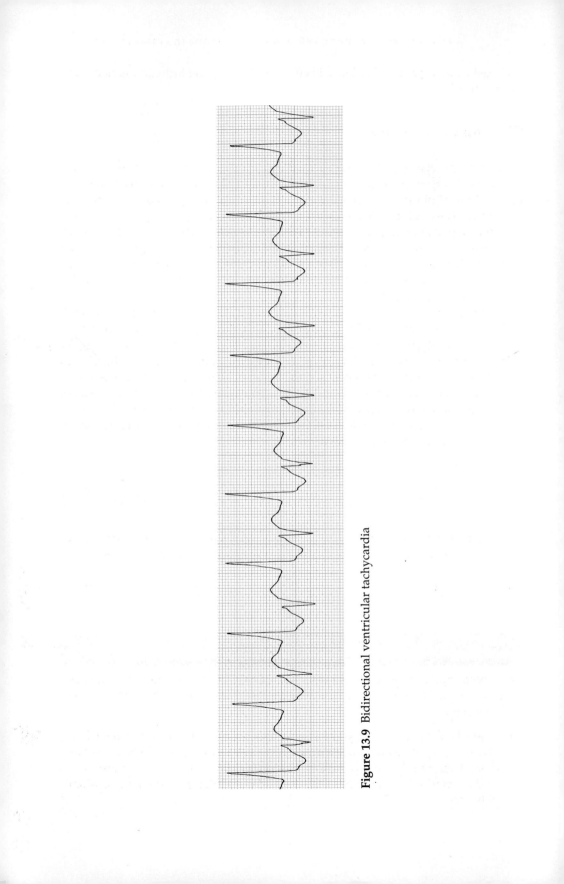

Figure 13.9 Bidirectional ventricular tachycardia

Occasionally a praecordial blow is effective. Usually defibrillation is necessary (*see* chapter 20).

BRUGADA SYNDROME

This syndrome has only been recognized in recent years. It is characterized by a typical ECG pattern of ST elevation in leads V1–V2 or V3, together with partial right bundle branch block, a structurally normal heart and a high risk of ventricular fibrillation. The QRS complex in lead V1 usually shows the most typical features: it ends with a positive component (akin to the J wave seen in hypothermia), followed by an elevated, down-sloping ST segment and negative T wave (Figure 13.7). The typical ECG abnormalities may be intermittent: intravenous flecainide or ajmaline will induce the typical pattern. Late potentials are often found and are a risk factor for ventricular fibrillation.

The condition is a genetically determined abnormality of a cardiac ion channel. It is due to an autosomal dominant gene. Not all patients give a family history of sudden cardiac death because commonly the condition arises by mutation.

Ventricular fibrillation can develop at any age, most commonly in middle life. No anti-arrhythmic drugs have been shown to be effective. The only treatment is implantation of an automatic defibrillator. Patients who have experienced syncope, have been resuscitated from ventricular fibrillation, have a strong family history of sudden cardiac death or have fibrillation induced at a ventricular stimulation study (Figure 13.8) should receive such a device.

BIDIRECTIONAL VENTRICULAR TACHYCARDIA

This is a rare arrhythmia with two alternating ventricular complex morphologies (Figure 13.9). It cannot be described as either monomorphic or polymorphic!

Main points

- Polymorphic tachycardia is characterized by repeated progressive changes in the QRS complex so the complexes appear to 'twist' about the baseline.

- Torsade de pointes tachycardia refers to polymorphic tachycardia when there is QT prolongation in between tachycardias. Casuses include bradycardia, a large number of drugs and the hereditary QT prolongation syndromes. Anti-arrhythmic therapy may aggravate the arrhythmia and pacing is often effective.

- Ventricular fibrillation is the rapid, totally incoordinate contraction of ventricular myocardial fibres. It causes circulatory arrest. The commonest cause is myocardial ischaemia. Rarely it will stop spontaneously, otherwise immediate defibrillation is necessary.

- The Brugada syndrome is a genetic disorder characterized by a specific pattern of ST elevation in the right praecordial leads and may result in sudden death from ventricular fibrillation.

CHAPTER 14

Tachycardias with broad ventricular complexes

Tachycardias of supraventricular origin sometimes have broad ventricular complexes. Thus, they may mimic ventricular tachycardia. Now that this is widely appreciated, the tendency is to misinterpret ventricular tachycardia as supraventricular, rather than the reverse.

CAUSES OF A BROAD COMPLEX TACHYCARDIA

Tachycardias with broad ventricular complexes can be due to:

1. ventricular tachycardia;
2. supraventricular tachycardia when bundle branch block has already been present during sinus rhythm;
3. supraventricular tachycardia with rate-related bundle branch block, i.e. bundle branch block develops during tachycardia;
4. the Wolff–Parkinson–White syndrome when atrial impulses during atrial flutter or fibrillation are conducted to the ventricles by the accessory AV pathway, or in the uncommon 'antidromic' form of AV re-entrant tachycardia when AV conduction is over the accessory pathway.

Several pointers are used to distinguish a supraventricular tachycardia with broad ventricular complexes from ventricular tachycardia.

USELESS GUIDELINES

It is often said that, whereas ventricular tachycardia leads to major haemodynamic disturbance, supraventricular tachycardia does not. This is wrong. Sometimes ventricular tachycardia causes few or even no symptoms, whereas supraventricular tachycardia, if very fast or in the presence of underlying heart disease, can cause shock or heart failure (Figure 14.1).

Another widely quoted but incorrect rule is that, whereas supraventricular tachycardia is regular, ventricular tachycardia is slightly irregular.

Verapamil may terminate supraventricular tachycardia or slow the ventricular response to atrial fibrillation or flutter. It has been used as a 'therapeutic' test of the origin of tachycardia. However, dangerous hypotension may result when the drug is given during ventricular tachycardia. Never use verapamil to try to establish the origin of a broad complex tachycardia.

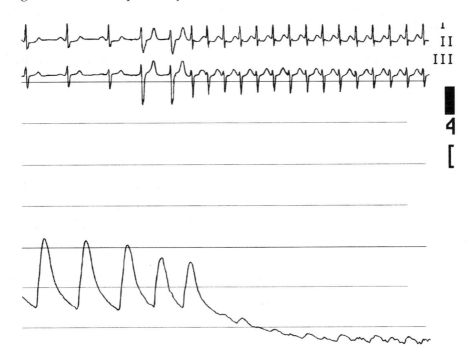

Figure 14.1 Dramatic drop in arterial pressure with onset of atrioventricular re-entrant tachycardia

USEFUL GUIDELINES

CLINICAL CIRCUMSTANCES

Myocardial damage caused by coronary artery disease, cardiomyopathy or by other diseases may cause ventricular tachycardia. On the other hand, myocardial damage is not going to create the additional electrical connection between atria and ventricles which is necessary to facilitate an AV re-entrant tachycardia. Thus, a broad QRS tachycardia in a patient known to have myocardial damage is likely to be ventricular in origin.

Atrial flutter and tachycardia may occur in patients with myocardial damage and may lead to a regular ventricular rhythm with bundle branch block but there are characteristic features which should lead to their identification. Atrial fibrillation is totally irregular and should never be confused with ventricular tachycardia.

INDEPENDENT ATRIAL ACTIVITY

If there is direct or indirect (Figures 12.2, 12.4, 12.10, 14.2 and 14.3) evidence of independent atrial activity, then supraventricular tachycardia is excluded. As discussed in chapter 5, scrutiny of several ECG leads may be necessary to identify evidence of atrial activity (Figure 14.4). Wherever possible, a 12-lead ECG during tachycardia should be acquired (Figure 14.5).

Occasionally, independent atrial activity can only be demonstrated by recording an atrial electrogram simultaneously with a surface ECG (Figure 14.6). An atrial electrogram can be obtained by passing a transvenous electrode to the right atrium or by using an oesophageal electrode positioned behind the left atrium.

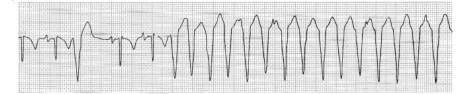

Figure 14.2 The second ventricular ectopic beat initiates ventricular tachycardia. Independent atrial activity can be seen

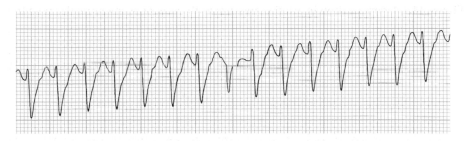

Figure 14.3 Ventricular tachycardia (lead II). The eighth complex is a capture beat

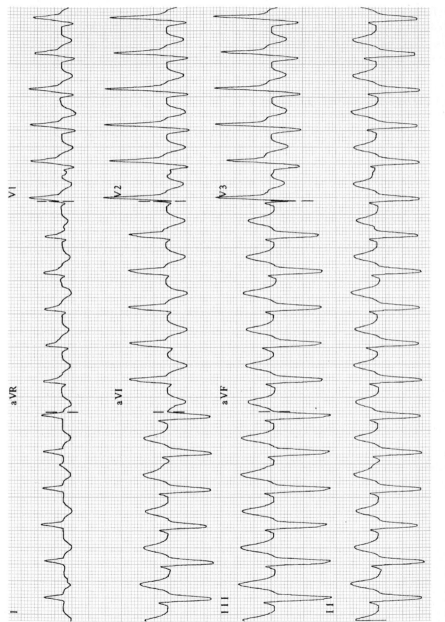
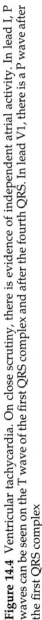

Figure 14.4 Ventricular tachycardia. On close scrutiny, there is evidence of independent atrial activity. In lead I, P waves can be seen on the T wave of the first QRS complex and after the fourth QRS. In lead V1, there is a P wave after the first QRS complex

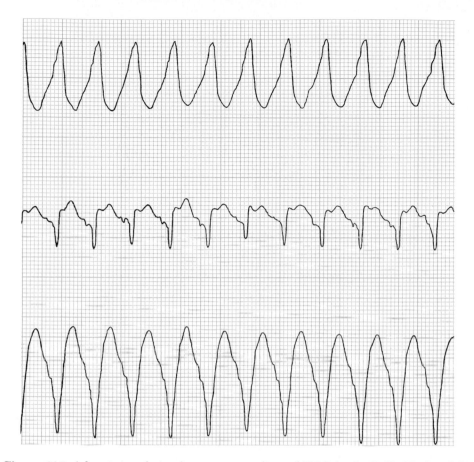

Figure 14.5 Advantage of simultaneous recording of ECG leads (I, II, III). Lead II suggests that there may be a P wave before each QRS complex and thus that the tachycardia is supraventricular in origin rather than ventricular. However, comparison with other leads indicates that the 'P' wave is in fact the initial vector of the ventricular complex

CAROTID SINUS MASSAGE

Carotid sinus massage can transiently slow AV node conduction and may thus terminate an AV re-entrant tachycardia. If a reduction in ventricular rate occurs during massage but sinus rhythm does not return, it is likely the patient has atrial flutter or fibrillation. During the higher degree of AV block, flutter and fibrillation waves are more easily identifiable. Carotid sinus massage is not always effective in supraventricular tachycardia and its failure does not indicate ventricular tachycardia.

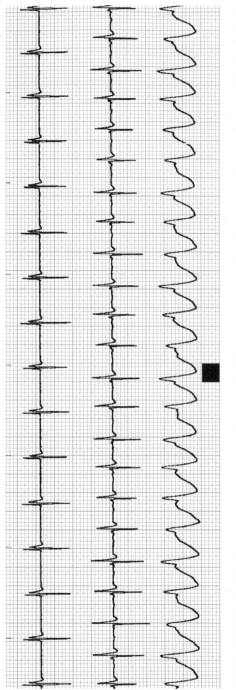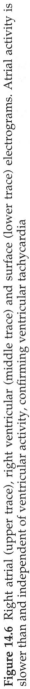

Figure 14.6 Right atrial (upper trace), right ventricular (middle trace) and surface (lower trace) electrograms. Atrial activity is slower than and independent of ventricular activity, confirming ventricular tachycardia

CONFIGURATION OF VENTRICULAR COMPLEX

The broader the ventricular complex, the more likely is a ventricular origin. In ventricular tachycardia, the duration of the ventricular complex is usually 0.14 s or greater.

Marked axis deviation, left or right, also suggests ventricular tachycardia. Another pointer towards this arrhythmia is a 'concordant' pattern in the chest leads, i.e. the complexes are either all positive or all negative (Figure 14.7).

When supraventricular tachycardias are associated with bundle branch block the morphology of the ventricular complexes is usually that of typical left or right bundle branch block.

RETROGRADE CONCEALED CONDUCTION

As discussed in chapter 2, partial penetration of the AV node by a ventricular ectopic impulse may lead to prolongation of the PR interval during the following sinus beat. Prolongation of the PR interval in the first sinus beat after a tachycardia indicates a ventricular origin.

ECTOPIC BEATS

If the configuration of the ventricular complex during tachycardia is similar to that of an ectopic beat recorded during normal rhythm, a common origin is probable. It is relatively easy to ascertain the origin of single ectopic beats, especially if a full ECG is available (Figure 14.2).

ADENOSINE

Adenosine is very effective at terminating supraventricular tachycardia due to an AV re-entrant mechanism and will transiently slow the ventricular response to atrial fibrillation and flutter, making the respective atrial 'f' or 'F' waves easily identifiable. A positive response to adenosine points strongly towards a supraventricular origin to the tachycardia. Because its duration of action is very brief, it is a safe drug to give (with the possible exception of patients with asthma).

However, a minority of supraventricular tachycardias will not respond to adenosine and the drug will terminate right ventricular outflow tract tachycardia. Thus response or lack of response to adenosine is a pointer towards the origin of the tachycardia but is not an absolutely reliable guide.

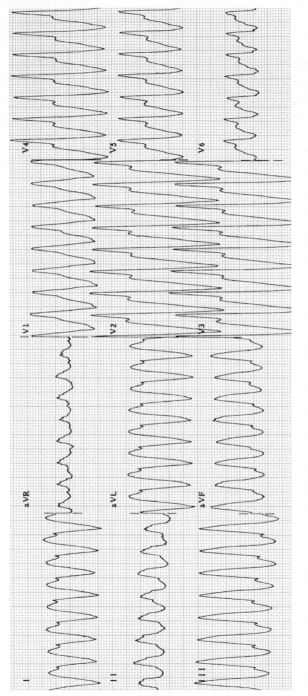

Figure 14.7 Ventricular tachycardia. QRS complex duration = 0.18 s. Concordant pattern in chest leads

Main points

- Wherever possible, record a 12-lead ECG during tachycardia.

- Though bundle branch block can sometimes occur during supraventricular tachycardias, most wide complex tachycardias are ventricular in origin.

- Pointers towards ventricular tachycardia include the presence of myocardial damage, direct or indirect evidence of independent atrial activity, QRS duration greater than 0.14 s, a concordant pattern in the chest leads and marked axis deviation.

- Neither minor irregularities during tachycardia or the haemodynamic effect of the arrhythmia are useful in ascertaining its origin.

- When supraventricular tachycardias are associated with bundle branch block the morphology of the ventricular complexes is usually that of typical left or right bundle branch block.

- Never use verapamil for a diagnostic test.

CHAPTER 15

Atrioventricular block

CLASSIFICATION

Atrioventricular block is classified as first, second or third degree depending on whether conduction of atrial impulses to the ventricles is delayed, intermittently blocked or completely blocked.

FIRST-DEGREE AV BLOCK

Delay in conduction of the atrial impulse to the ventricles results in prolongation of the PR interval (Figures 15.1–15.3). The PR interval is measured from the onset of the P wave to the onset of the ventricular complex – whether this be a Q or an R wave – and is prolonged if it is greater than 0.21 s.

First-degree AV block does not cause symptoms but may sometimes progress to higher degrees of block. In young people it is usually due to high vagal tone and is benign.

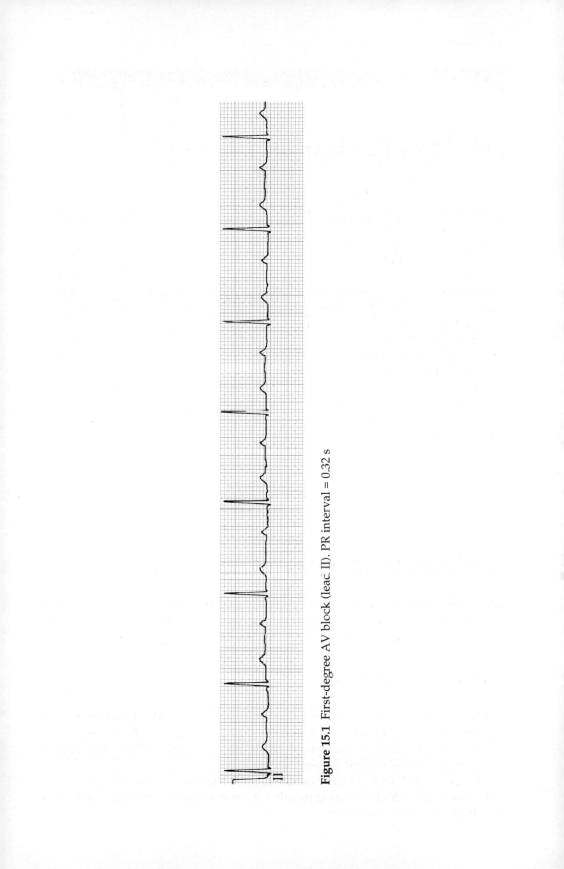

Figure 15.1 First-degree AV block (lead II). PR interval = 0.32 s

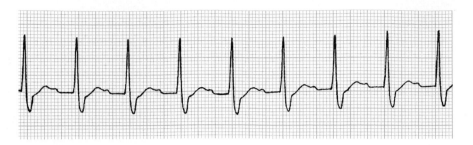

Figure 15.2 First-degree AV block and sinus tachycardia (lead I). PR interval = 0.24 s

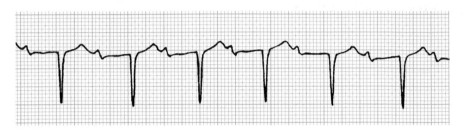

Figure 15.3 First-degree AV block (lead V1). The P wave is superimposed on the terminal portion of the preceding T wave. PR interval = 0.38 s

SECOND-DEGREE AV BLOCK

In second-degree AV block there is intermittent failure of conduction of atrial impulses to the ventricles, i.e. P waves not followed by QRS complexes. Second-degree block is subdivided into Mobitz type I (which is also termed 'Wenkebach') and Mobitz type II block.

Mobitz type I or Wenkebach AV block

In this form of second-degree block, delay in AV conduction increases with each successive atrial impulse until an atrial impulse fails to be conducted to the ventricles. After the dropped beat, AV conduction recovers and the sequence starts again (Figures 15.4 and 15.5).

AV Wenkebach block is usually due to impaired conduction in the AV node. Like first-degree AV block, it can be benign (particularly during sleep) and is due to high vagal tone. Recent evidence suggests that Wenkebach block which cannot be attributed to high vagal tone has a similar prognosis to Mobitz II block.

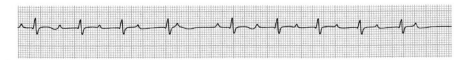

Figure 15.4 AV Wenkebach block

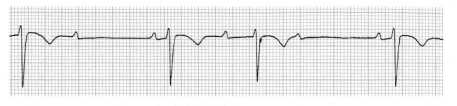

Figure 15.5 AV Wenkebach block. Unlike many textbook examples, but as often occurs in practice, the trace does not start with the shortest PR interval

Mobitz type II AV block

In Mobitz type II block there is intermittent failure of conduction of atrial impulses to the ventricles without preceding progressive lengthening of the PR interval, and thus the PR interval of conducted beats is constant (Figure 15.6).

In contrast to first-degree and Wenkebach AV block, Mobitz type II block is usually due to impaired conduction in the bundle of His or bundle branches, i.e. infranodal. Thus, because there is bundle branch disease, the QRS complexes are usually broad. Block below the AV node is more likely to be associated with Stokes–Adams attacks, slow ventricular rates and sudden death.

The ratio of conducted to nonconducted atrial impulses varies. Commonly 2:1 AV conduction occurs (Figure 15.7). A similar pattern may be caused by an extreme

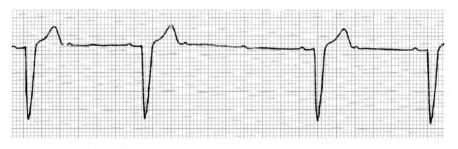

Figure 15.6 Mobitz type II AV block. In this example the ratio between conducted and nonconducted atrial impulses varies

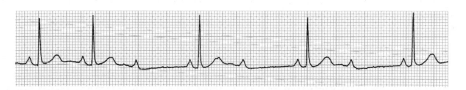

Figure 15.7 After two normally conducted beats there is Mobitz type II AV block with 2:1 AV conduction

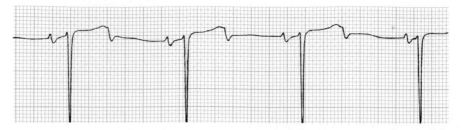

Figure 15.8 2:1 AV block with narrow QRS complexes (lead V1). The nonconducted atrial beats are superimposed on preceding T waves

form of Wenkebach block so it is difficult to make prognostic inferences from 2:1 AV block with narrow QRS complexes (Figure 15.8).

Usually, during Mobitz type II block, the atrial rate is regular. Sometimes, however, the P–P interval encompassing a ventricular complex is shorter than a P–P interval which does not. This is known as ventriculophasic sinus arrhythmia.

THIRD-DEGREE AV BLOCK

Third-degree or complete AV block occurs when there is total interruption of transmission of atrial impulses to the ventricles. Third-degree block may be due to interrupted conduction at either AV nodal or infranodal level. When the block is within the AV node, subsidiary pacemakers arise within the bundle of His and, unless there is additional bundle branch block, will lead to narrow QRS complexes (Figure 15.9). Often, pacemakers within the bundle of His discharge reliably at a fairly rapid rate. In contrast, in infranodal block subsidiary pacemakers usually arise in the left or right bundle branches. These pacemakers will produce broad QRS complexes and slower ventricular rates (Figures 15.10 and 15.13). They are less reliable and thus Stokes–Adams attacks are more likely.

Complete AV block can complicate atrial fibrillation and flutter (Figures 15.11 and 15.12).

Occasionally, heart block only occurs during exercise and can be the cause of exertional syncope or weakness.

Supernormal conduction

Occasionally, even during third-degree AV block, atrial impulses may be conducted to the ventricles. There is a short period immediately after recovery from excitation when AV conduction may transiently improve. This period usually coincides with inscription of the latter portion of the T wave (Figure 15.13). As a result, atrial impulses falling on this part of the T wave will be followed by a premature QRS complex.

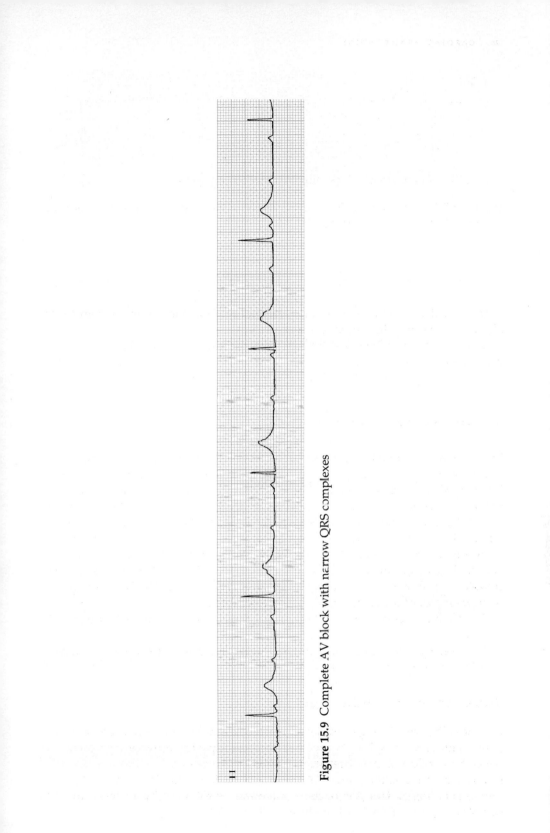

Figure 15.9 Complete AV block with narrow QRS complexes

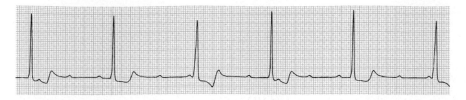

Figure 15.10 Complete AV block with broad QRS complexes

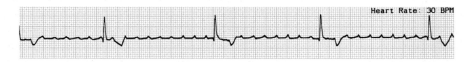

Figure 15.11 Complete AV block with atrial fibrillation

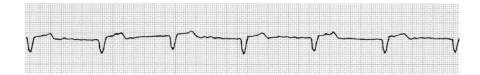

Figure 15.12 Complete AV block with atrial flutter

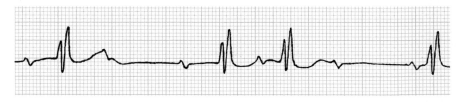

Figure 15.13 Complete AV block. There is supernormal conduction of the atrial impulse that falls on the T wave of the second ventricular complex (lead V1)

CAUSES OF AV BLOCK

Idiopathic fibrosis of the AV junction and/or bundle branches is the most common cause. The causes of AV block are listed in Table 15.1.

Table 15.1 Causes of atrioventricular block

Idiopathic fibrosis of conduction tissues
Myocardial infarction
Aortic valve disease
Congenital isolated lesion
Congenital heart disease, e.g. corrected transposition
Cardiac surgery
Infiltration, e.g. tumour, sarcoidosis, haemochromatosis, syphilis
Inflammation, e.g. endocarditis, ankylosing spondylitis, Reiter's syndrome
Rheumatic fever
Diphtheria
Dystrophia myotonica
Chagas' disease (South America)
Lyme carditis (tick-borne spirochaetal infection, *Borrelia burgdorferi*, mainly North America)

AV DISSOCIATION

During third-degree AV block, atrial activity is faster than and dissociated from ventricular activity. Dissociation between atrial and ventricular activity also occurs when, often during sinus bradycardia, an escape rhythm faster than the sinus rate arises from the AV junction or ventricles (Figure 15.14). The term 'AV dissociation' should be reserved for this latter situation, in which the ventricular rate is greater than the atrial rate. If AV dissociation is not distinguished from complete AV block, inappropriate action can result. For example, AV dissociation often occurs in acute myocardial infarction and, if not recognized as such, a pacemaker may be unnecessarily inserted.

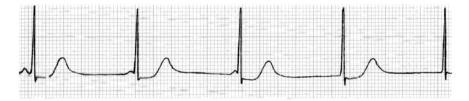

Figure 15.14 AV dissociation. Atrial and ventricular rates are 49 and 51 beats/min, respectively. The fourth and fifth P waves are concealed by superimposed QRS complexes

BILATERAL BUNDLE BRANCH DISEASE

Infranodal AV block is most often caused by disease in both left and right bundle branches.

Although the anatomical situation may be more complex, functionally the bundle of His can be considered to divide into three: the right bundle branch and the anterior and posterior fascicles of the left bundle branch (*see* chapter 4).

If conduction is blocked in only two of the three fascicles (bifascicular block), the functioning fascicle will conduct atrial impulses to the ventricles and maintain sinus rhythm. Block in the third fascicle will lead to complete AV block.

Bifascicular block

The most common pattern of bifascicular block is right bundle branch plus left anterior fascicular block (Figure 15.15). The posterior fascicle of the left bundle branch is a stouter structure than the anterior fascicle and is therefore less vulnerable. As a result, right bundle branch plus left posterior fascicular block is a less common occurrence (Figure 15.16).

PR interval prolongation is usually due to impaired AV node conduction, but in the context of bifascicular block it is more likely to reflect abnormal conduction in the functioning fascicle (Figure 15.17).

Trifascicular block

Interrupted conduction in all three fascicles results in complete AV block. In many patients one of the three fascicles is capable of intermittent conduction so that, for part of the time, there will be sinus rhythm with evidence of bifascicular block.

The risk of bifascicular block progressing to trifascicular block is low. In patients with right bundle and left anterior fascicular block, it is a few per cent per year. The risk is increased when there is right bundle and left posterior fascicular block and when there is alternating complete right and left bundle branch block. There is little evidence to suggest that prophylactic implantation of a permanent pacemaker in asymptomatic patients with bifascicular block improves prognosis. The major determinants of prognosis are the states of the myocardium and coronary arteries.

CLINICAL FEATURES OF AV BLOCK

First-degree and Mobitz type I second-degree AV block do not cause symptoms but may progress to higher grades of block.

In Mobitz type II and complete AV block, a low ventricular rate may cause tiredness, dyspnoea or heart failure. In some patients the ventricular pacemaker may at times discharge very slowly or actually stop, leading to syncope or, if ventricular activity does not quickly return, sudden death (Figure 15.18). Ventricular fibrillation and tachycardia arise in some patients as a consequence of the low ventricular rate and may also lead to syncope or sudden death.

Stokes–Adams attacks

Syncope due to transient asystole or ventricular tachyarrhyhmia – a Stokes–Adams attack – has characteristic features. These features are of great diagnostic importance.

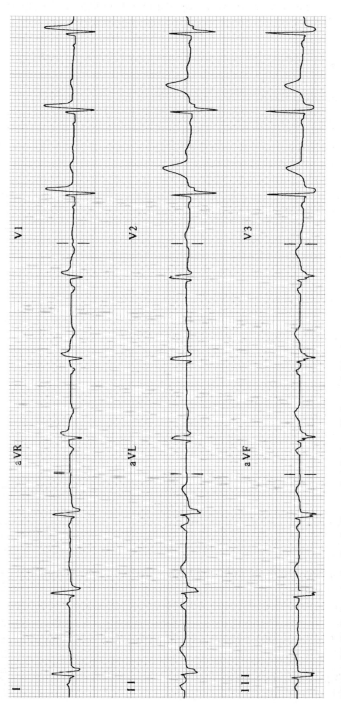

Figure 15.15 Left anterior fascicular and right bundle branch block

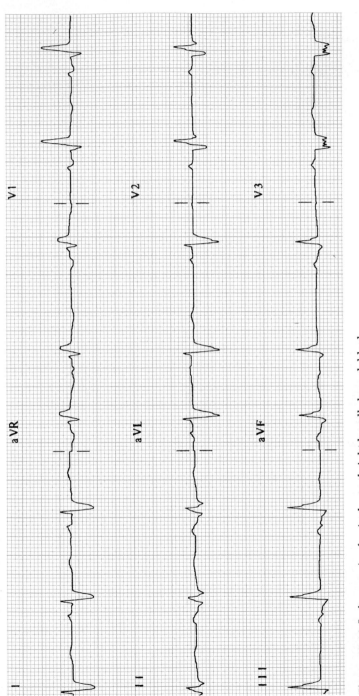

Figure 15.16 Left posterior fascicular and right bundle branch block

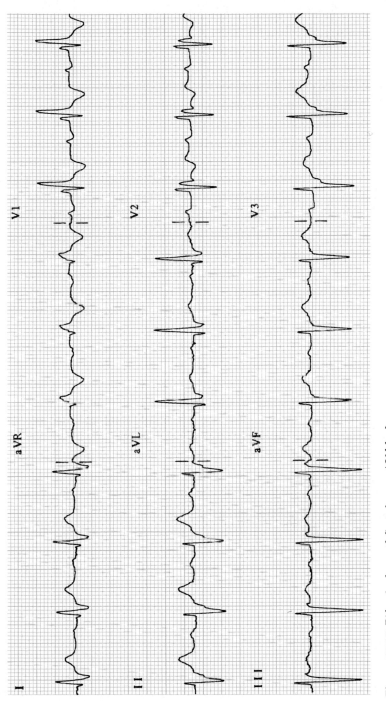

Figure 15.17 Bifascicular and first-degree AV block

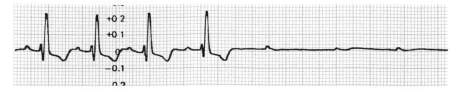

Figure 15.18 Sudden onset of complete AV block with no escape rhythm in a patient with bifascicular block

On the one hand, abnormalities of AV conduction (and sinus node function) may be intermittent, routine electrocardiography being normal, and on the other hand, in patients with evidence of disease of the specialized conducting tissues, syncope may occasionally be due to unrelated causes such as epilepsy.

In a Stokes–Adams attack, loss of consciousness is sudden. There is virtually no warning, though the patient will sometimes feel that he is going to faint, just before he loses consciousness. The patient collapses, lying motionless, pale and pulseless. He looks as though he or she is dead. Usually, within a minute or two, consciousness returns, and as cardiac action resumes there may be a vivid flush to the skin. Incontinence does occur occasionally but is not a regular feature as it is in epilepsy. Unlike epilepsy, recovery is quick, and confusion and headache after the attack are unusual.

NEAR-SYNCOPE

In some patients the rhythm disturbance does not last long enough to cause syncope but the patient feels as though he or she is going to faint and then recovers. The patient may complain of 'dizziness' but will not experience true vertigo.

CONGENITAL HEART BLOCK

AV conduction is interrupted at the AV nodal level. Consequently, the subsidiary ventricular pacemaker is situated in the proximal part of the bundle of His (producing narrow QRS complexes) and discharges reliably at a moderately fast rate (40–80 beats/min), which may accelerate on exercise. Often, there are no symptoms and exercise tolerance is good. However, syncope and sudden death do occur in a minority of patients (*see* chapter 24).

ACQUIRED HEART BLOCK

Heart block complicating myocardial infarction is discussed in chapter 18.

As discussed above, the commonest cause of heart block is idiopathic fibrosis of the AV junction or bundle branches. This mainly affects the elderly but – as with the other causes of AV block – it can affect the young and middle aged as well.

The bradycardia associated with Mobitz type II and third-degree AV block may reduce cardiac output and lead to symptoms such as shortness of breath, tiredness and heart failure. Stokes–Adams attacks will sooner or later occur in about two-thirds of patients with these higher grades of AV block.

TREATMENT

Artificial cardiac pacing has greatly improved symptoms and prognosis. The indications are discussed in chapters 23 and 24.

Main points

- AV block is classified as first, second or third degree depending on whether conduction of atrial impulses to the ventricles is delayed, intermittently blocked or completely blocked.

- Second-degree AV block is subdivided into Mobitz I (Wenkebach) and Mobitz II types. In the former, there is progressive lengthening of the PR interval prior to nonconduction of an atrial impulse, whereas the PR interval of conducted atrial impulses is constant in Mobitz II.

- During AV dissociation (in contrast to complete AV block), the atrial rate is slower than the ventricular rate.

- First-degree block, Wenkebach block and third-degree block with narrow QRS complexes are usually due to disease within the AV node, whereas Mobitz II and complete block with broad QRS complexes are likely to be due to infranodal block.

- Bifascicular block may deteriorate intermittently or permanently to complete (trifascicular) AV block.

- Stokes–Adams attacks are characterized by abrupt loss of consciousness which lasts for a few minutes only, following which recovery is usually rapid. Patients with conduction tissue disease often experience 'near-syncope' as well as episodes of complete loss of consciousness.

CHAPTER 16

Sick sinus syndrome

The sick sinus syndrome, which is also referred to as sino-atrial disease, is caused by impairment of either sinus node automaticity or of conduction of impulses from the sinus node to the atria. It can lead to sinus bradycardia, sino-atrial block or sinus arrest.

In some patients, atrial fibrillation, flutter or tachycardia may also occur. The term 'bradycardia–tachycardia' (often shortened to 'brady–tachy') syndrome applies to these patients.

Sick sinus syndrome is a common cause of syncope, dizzy attacks and palpitation. Though found most often in the elderly, it can occur at any age.

CAUSES

The cause is usually idiopathic fibrosis of the sinus node. Cardiomyopathy, myocarditis, cardiac surgery and anti-arrhythmic drugs can also cause the syndrome.

ECG CHARACTERISTICS

Any of the following can occur. They are often intermittent, normal sinus rhythm being present for most of the time.

Sinus bradycardia

Sinus bradycardia is a common finding (Figure 16.1).

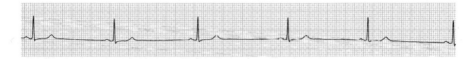

Figure 16.1 Sinus bradycardia: rate 33 beats/min

Sinus arrest

Sinus arrest is due to failure of the sinus node to activate the atria. The result is absence of normal P waves (Figures 16.2 and 16.3).

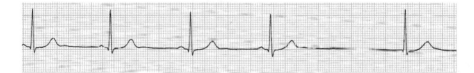

Figure 16.2 Sinus arrest leading to a junctional escape beat

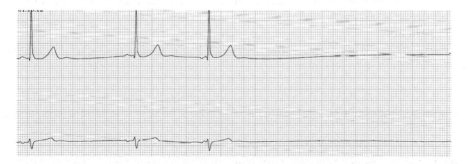

Figure 16.3 Sinus arrest after a junctional beat leading to a prolonged period of ventricular standstill

SINO-ATRIAL BLOCK

Sino-atrial block occurs when sinus node impulses fail to traverse the junction between the node and surrounding atrial myocardium. Like atrioventricular block, sino-atrial block can be classified into first, second or third degrees. However, the ECG allows only recognition of second-degree sino-atrial block. Third-degree or complete block is indistinguishable from sinus arrest.

In second-degree sino-atrial block, intermittent failure of atrial activation results in intervals between P waves which are multiples of (often twice) the cycle length during sinus rhythm (Figure 16.4).

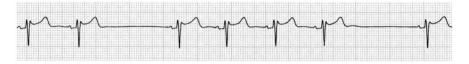

Figure 16.4 Two pauses due to second-degree sino-atrial block during which both the P waves and QRS complexes are dropped for one cycle

ESCAPE BEATS AND RHYTHMS

When sinus bradycardia or arrest occurs, subsidiary pacemaker tissue may give rise to an escape beat or rhythm (Figures 16.2 and 16.5). A junctional or idioventricular rhythm suggests impaired sinus node function.

ATRIAL ECTOPIC BEATS

These are common. Long pauses often follow because sinus node automaticity is depressed by the ectopic beat (Figure 16.6).

BRADYCARDIA–TACHYCARDIA SYNDROME

Atrial fibrillation, flutter or tachycardia may occur in patients with sick sinus syndrome (Figure 16.7). However, AV re-entrant tachycardia is not part of this syndrome.

Sinus node automaticity is often depressed by these tachycardias, so sinus brady-cardia or arrest follows the tachycardia. Conversely, tachycardias often arise as an escape rhythm during bradycardia. Thus, tachycardia often alternates with brady-cardia (Figure 16.8).

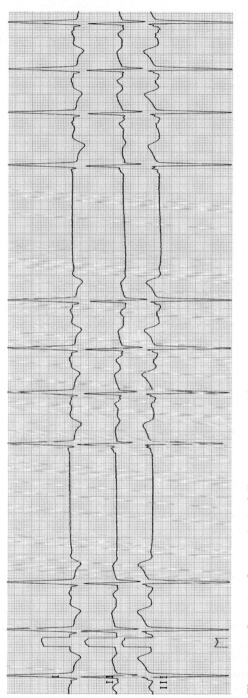

Figure 16.5 Junctional escape beats following sinus arrest

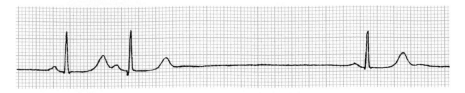

Figure 16.6 Atrial ectopic beat leads to depression of sinus node automaticity

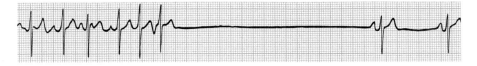

Figure 16.7 Termination of atrial fibrillation followed by sinus arrest

AV BLOCK

AV block sometimes coexists with sick sinus syndrome.

In patients with sick sinus syndrome who develop atrial fibrillation there is often a slow ventricular response without AV nodal-blocking drugs suggesting co-existent impaired AV nodal function.

CLINICAL FEATURES

Sinus arrest without an adequate escape rhythm may cause syncope or dizzy attacks, depending on its duration. Tachycardias often produce palpitation, and resultant sinus node depression may lead to syncope or near-syncope after palpitation.

Some patients will experience symptoms several times each day, whereas in others symptoms will be infrequent.

Systemic embolism is common in the bradycardia–tachycardia syndrome.

DIAGNOSIS

Suspect sick sinus syndrome when there is syncope, near-syncope or palpitation in the presence of sinus bradycardia or an escape rhythm. Prolonged sinus arrest or sino-atrial block confirms the diagnosis.

Sometimes the standard ECG will provide diagnostic information but often ambulatory electrocardiography will be necessary.

Sinus bradycardia and short pauses during sleep are normal and are not evidence for the sick sinus syndrome. Furthermore, pauses in sinus node activity of up to 2.0 s due to high vagal tone may be found in fit, young people.

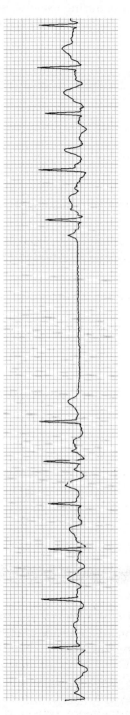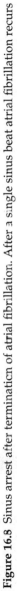

Figure 16.8 Sinus arrest after termination of atrial fibrillation. After a single sinus beat atrial fibrillation recurs

A 24-h tape recording in a normal subject will inevitably show sinus bradycardia during sleep and sinus tachycardia during exercise. Sometimes these are wrongly taken as evidence of the bradycardia–tachycardia syndrome!

TREATMENT

SINUS BRADYCARDIA OR ARREST

Cardiac pacing is necessary to control symptoms (*see* chapter 24).

For two reasons, atrial pacing, which preserves the normal sequence of cardiac chamber activation, is preferable to ventricular pacing. Ventricular pacing may result in the pacemaker syndrome and atrial systole lessens the risk of systemic embolism.

An AV sequential pacemaker is required if there is AV or bundle branch block or if at implantation, atrial pacing at 120 beats/min causes AV block.

BRADYCARDIA–TACHYCARDIA SYNDROME

Anti-arrhythmic drugs often worsen sinus node function. A pacemaker is usually necessary if drugs are needed to control tachycardias.

Tachycardias often arise during sinus bradycardia or pauses. Atrial pacing may well prevent tachyarrhythmias.

The risk of systemic embolism is high. Anticoagulation is indicated unless tachy-arrhythmias can be prevented.

Main points

- The sick sinus syndrome is due to impaired sinus node function or sino-atrial conduction and may cause sinus bradycardia, sino-atrial block or sinus arrest.

- A long pause in sinus node activity without an adequate junctional or ventricular escape rhythm will cause near-syncope or syncope.

- The bradycardia–tachycardia syndrome is the association of sinus node dysfunction with episodes of atrial fibrillation, flutter or tachycardia (but not atrioventricular re-entrant tachycardia). There is a high risk of systemic embolism.

- Artificial cardiac pacing is required for control of symptoms and to prevent bradycardia if anti-arrhythmic drugs are to be prescribed for the bradycardia–tachycardia syndrome.

CHAPTER 17

Neurally mediated syncope

This term refers to carotid sinus syndrome, malignant vasovagal syncope and less common syndromes such as micturition syncope in which triggering of an autonomic nervous system reflex results in syncope due to inappropriate vaso-dilatation and/or bradycardia.

Neurally mediated syncope should be considered in patients with unexplained syncope without electrocardiographic evidence of sick sinus syndrome or AV block.

CAROTID SINUS SYNDROME

The diagnosis of carotid sinus syndrome is made in patients who suffer from near-syncope or syncope in whom unilateral carotid sinus massage for 5–10 s causes sinus arrest or complete AV block for 3 s or more (Figure 17.1). In some patients, severe hypotension due to vasodilation (vasodepression) occurs as well as brady-cardia (cardioinhibition).

In contrast to syncope caused by sick sinus syndrome or AV block, loss of consciousness may be prolonged due to persistent hypotension, and fitting and incontinence can occur.

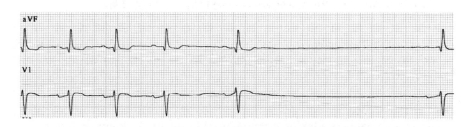

Figure 17.1 Carotid sinus syndrome. Carotid sinus massage causes 3 s sinus arrest

Cardiac pacing (*see* chapter 24) will improve or abolish symptoms. However, in some patients, the vasodepressor element continues to cause symptoms in spite of pacing.

Some asymptomatic subjects, particularly among the elderly, may develop a marked bradycardia on carotid massage. Carotid sinus syndrome should only be diagnosed in patients with typical spontaneous symptoms.

MALIGNANT VASOVAGAL SYNDROME

The term 'malignant' is used to distinguish this syndrome from vasovagal syncope or faint commonly seen in young people. With the former, there are no prodromal symptoms or triggering factors such as pain or the sight of blood.

The syndrome is characterized by recurrent, abrupt syncope, when sitting or standing, and a positive tilt table test. Results from other usual tests used to investigate syncope are negative. The risk of death is very low. Frequency of recurrence of attacks is variable and unpredictable.

Syncope is thought to result from pooling of blood in the lower extremeties. Reduced venous return leads to hypotension. This is detected by baroreceptors and leads to enhanced sympathetic nervous system activity and thus increased force of myocardial contraction. Because of reduced venous return, the left ventricle is relatively empty. Systole results in excessive stimulation of ventricular mechano-receptors which trigger inappropriate reflex vasodilatation and bradycardia. Reflex control of venous tone has also been shown to be abnormal. In some patients 'cardioinhibtion', i.e. bradycardia, either sinus arrest or AV block, predominates while in others it is the 'vasodepressor' element, i.e. vasodilatation which is the main prolem.

Tilt table test

The patient is gently secured on a tilt table and rapidly tilted from the supine position to a 60 degree angle, standing on a footplate, for up to 45 minutes. The ECG and blood pressure are continuously monitored. The test is positive if syncope results from profound bradycardia (often asystole) and/or hypotension (Figures 17.2 and 17.3). A positive result rarely occurs in normal subjects. Drugs such as isoprenaline and glyceryl trinitrate are sometimes used to provoke syncope.

Treatment

Patients should be advised to avoid situations which encourage venous pooling. They should avoid standing or sitting for prolonged periods and should regularly contract the muscles in their legs to aid venous return. Dehydration should also be avoided.

Dual-chamber cardiac pacing is indicated to treat the cardioinhibitory element of the syndrome in patients who have experienced frequent blackouts. Because pacing will not prevent the vasodepressor element of the syndrome, symptoms may

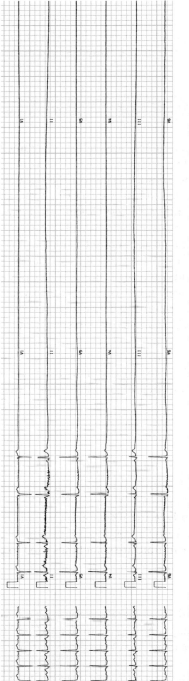

Figure 17.2 Malignant vasovagal syndrome. Asystole and then fitting developed after 3 min on a tilt table

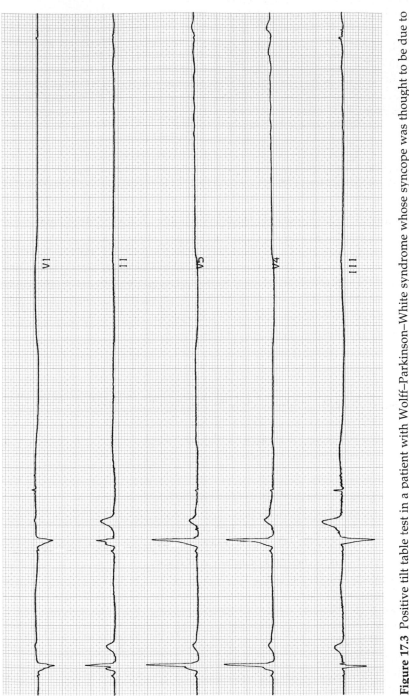

Figure 17.3 Positive tilt table test in a patient with Wolff–Parkinson–White syndrome whose syncope was thought to be due to paroxysmal tachycardia

continue. In general, pacing will reduce the frequency and severity of symptoms but only a minority will be rendered symptom free.

A rate drop algorithm is probably the best method of pacing for patients with the malignant vasovagal syndrome; a sudden reduction in heart rate will trigger pacing at a high rate: 90–130 beats/min. The high rate may compensate for the vaso-depressor effect.

Treatment of the vasodepressor component is difficult. A number of drugs have been tried: beta-blockers, disopyramide, scopolamine skin patches, midodrine and fludrocortisone. None have been shown to be very effective.

SIMPLE FAINT

Syncope due to the malignant vasovagal syndrome must be distinguished from the 'simple' faint which is common in young people. This is triggered by a variety of 'situational factors' such as unpleasant sights (e.g. sight of blood or needles), pain, extreme emotion and stuffy rooms. Common places for fainting are churches, hospitals, and restaurants. In contrast to the malignant vasovagal syndrome where syncope is of abrupt onset, there is a history of preceding dizziness, sweating and nausea prior to loss of consciousness. Witnesses often report marked pallor. Weakness and nausea usually occur during recovery.

CAUSES OF SYNCOPE

When a patient presents with syncope it is important to bear in mind the many possible causes which are listed below.

- Cardiac arrhythmias:
  - sinus node disease;
  - atrioventricular block;
  - paroxysmal supraventricular tachycardia;
  - paroxysmal ventricular tachycardia or fibrillation, including hereditary long QT syndromes and Brugada syndrome.
- Neurally mediated syncope:
  - simple, common faint;
  - carotid sinus syndrome;
  - malignant vasovagal syndrome.
- Structural heart disease:
  - aortic stenosis;
  - hypertrophic cardiomyopathy;
  - atrial myxoma;
  - acute myocardial ischaemia;
  - pulmonary embolism.

- Orthostatic hypotension:
  - disorders of autonomic nervous syndrome – primary and caused by diabetes, amyloidosis;
  - haemorrhage;
  - diarrhoea;
  - Addison's disease.

Main points

- Carotid sinus and malignant vasovagal syndromes are caused by abnormal autonomic nervous system reflexes and can cause syncope due to bradycardia and or hypotension.

- The malignant vasovagal syndrome is characterized by recurrent, abrupt syncope, when sitting or standing, and a positive tilt table test.

- Tilt table testing can be used to demonstrate the cardioinhibitory and/or vasodepressor elements of the malignant vasovagal syndrome. Pacing may prevent or reduce syncope when caused by the former but will not influence symptoms due to the latter.

Arrhythmias due to myocardial infarction

Myocardial infarction causes a wide variety of arrhythmias (Table 18.1). Some require immediate action, whereas no treatment is necessary for others. Arrhythmias are most frequent in the early hours after infarction.

Table 18.1 Incidence of arrhythmias in a series of patients within 4 hours of myocardial infarction

Ventricular fibrillation	16%
Ventricular tachycardia	4%
Ventricular ectopic beats	93%
Supraventricular arrhythmias	6%
Sinus or junctional bradycardia	34%
Second- or third-degree AV block	7%

VENTRICULAR FIBRILLATION

Ninety per cent of deaths caused by myocardial infarction are due to ventricular fibrillation. The incidence of fibrillation is highest in the first hour after the onset of chest pain and decreases progressively thereafter. Forty per cent of deaths occur within the first hour. Thus many patients die before they can be admitted to hospital.

In those patients who reach hospital, however, ventricular fibrillation and other arrhythmias are sufficiently common to necessitate continuous ECG monitoring for 24–48 h in an area where facilities for resuscitation are immediately available, i.e. a coronary care unit. Between 3% and 10% of patients with acute myocardial infarction develop ventricular fibrillation while in a coronary care unit. The shorter the delay before admission, the greater is the incidence of ventricular fibrillation.

Ventricular fibrillation is most often initiated by an 'R on T' ventricular ectopic beat (Figure 18.1).

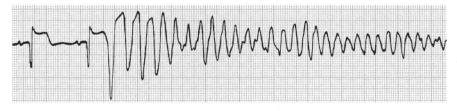

Figure 18.1 Ventricular ectopic beat initiating ventricular fibrillation

OTHER CAUSES

Ventricular fibrillation can also occur late after infarction and, in patients with severe coronary artery disease, without myocardial infarction, it may be the first clinical manifestation of the disease.

PRIMARY AND SECONDARY VENTRICULAR FIBRILLATION

If ventricular fibrillation develops in a heart that was functioning satisfactorily during normal rhythm, it is termed 'primary' fibrillation, whereas if it occurs in the context of cardiac failure or cardiogenic shock, it is termed 'secondary'. Successful defibrillation is less likely in secondary ventricular fibrillation.

TREATMENT

Rarely ventricular fibrillation is a brief event, spontaneously reverting to normal rhythm. Otherwise, without prompt treatment, irreversible cerebral and myocardial damage will quickly ensue.

Occasionally, a praecordial blow is effective but usually defibrillation is necessary (*see* chapter 20). On a coronary care unit, a defibrillator should be immediately available so little or no time need be spent on cardiopulmonary resuscitation.

A 200 J shock will successfully defibrillate 90% of cases. If unsuccessful, a second shock at the same energy level may be effective. The energy of a further shock should be increased to 360 J. The treatment of resistant ventricular fibrillation is discussed in chapter 21.

Following restoration of normal rhythm, an infusion of lignocaine is usually given to prevent further ventricular fibrillation, though there is little evidence to show that lignocaine or other anti-arrhythmic drugs are effective in this situation.

Ventricular flutter

Ventricular flutter is a very rapid ventricular rhythm in which there are continuous changes in waveform, distinction between QRS complexes and T waves being impossible (Figure 18.2). For practical purposes, it is the same as ventricular fibrillation.

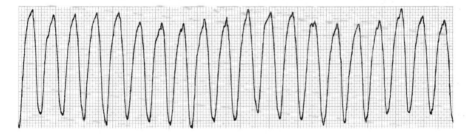

Figure 18.2 Ventricular flutter

Prevention of ventricular fibrillation in acute infarction

Conventional teaching used to be that ventricular ectopic beats which were frequent, multifocal, 'R on T', or repetitive – the 'warning arrhythmias' – heralded ventricular fibrillation or tachycardia (Figures 18.3–18.6). It was common practice to suppress these ectopic beats with anti-arrhythmic agents.

However, analysis of continuous ECG recordings has shown ventricular ectopic beats occur in almost all cases of acute infarction and warning arrhythmias are as common in patients who do not develop ventricular fibrillation as in those who do. Furthermore, warning arrhythmias may not precede ventricular fibrillation and, when these do occur, staff in even the best coronary care units often fail to detect them.

Since 'warning arrhythmias' do not in fact warn, it has been advocated that all patients should receive lignocaine. Several recent studies in the 'thrombolytic era'

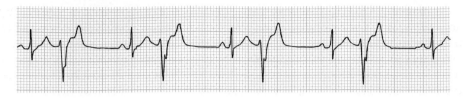

Figure 18.3 Frequent unifocal ventricular ectopic beats

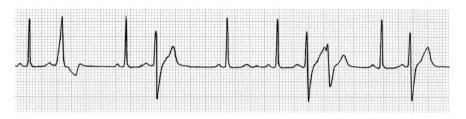

Figure 18.4 Frequent multifocal ventricular ectopic beats. The first ectopic beat arises from a different focus from that of subsequent ectopic beats. There is a couplet of ectopic beats after the fourth sinus beat

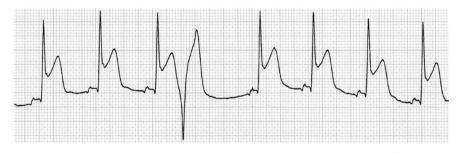

Figure 18.5 'R on T' ventricular ectopic beat

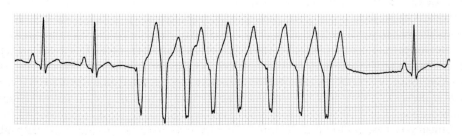

Figure 18.6 Salvo of ventricular ectopic beats

have shown that lignocaine does reduce the incidence of ventricular fibrillation by about 30% but mortality from acute infarction is not reduced; in fact, a trend to increased mortality has been shown. Furthermore, these studies have shown that, even though thrombolysis may sometimes cause ventricular fibrillation (a reperfusion arrhythmia), the overall incidence of ventricular fibrillation is low. The current consensus is that prophylactic lignocaine is not advisable.

Oral mexiletine, a drug similar to lignocaine, has been shown to increase mortality in acute infarction.

VENTRICULAR TACHYCARDIA

Ventricular tachycardia may be self-terminating (Figure 18.6) or sustained (Figure 18.7). Ventricular tachycardia may be initiated by either 'R on T' or later ventricular ectopic beats (Figure 18.8).

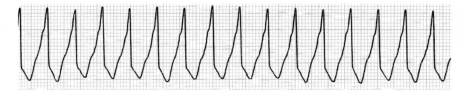

Figure 18.7 Monomorphic ventricular tachycardia

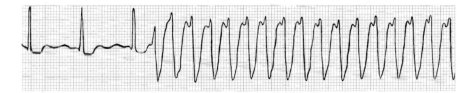

Figure 18.8 Ventricular tachycardia initiated by 'R on T' ectopic beat

Sometimes ventricular tachycardia will result in shock or circulatory arrest. On the other hand, ventricular tachycardia may cause few or no symptoms. In myocardial infarction a regular tachycardia with broad ventricular complexes is usually ventricular in origin, even in the absence of haemodynamic deterioration.

Nonsustained ventricular tachycardia is very common in the first 24 h following acute infarction. Only sustained ventricular tachycardia requires treatment. If cardiac arrest or shock occurs, immediate synchronized cardioversion (*see* chapter 20) is necessary. Otherwise intravenous lignocaine should be given. If lignocaine fails, second-line drugs include sotalol and amiodarone. Cardioversion may be necessary if a second-line drug fails. Overdrive ventricular pacing may help in recurrent ventricular tachycardia.

LONG-TERM SIGNIFICANCE OF VENTRICULAR ARRHYTHMIAS

Ventricular tachycardia and fibrillation within the first 24 h of myocardial infarction are unlikely to recur after that period. Thus anti-arrhythmic therapy after discharge from the coronary care unit is unnecessary. While most studies suggest early ventricular arrhythmias are not related to the amount of myocardial damage and are not of long-term prognostic significance, there are studies that suggest that early primary ventricular fibrillation is associated with an impaired prognosis and may be a mark of extensive infarction (Table 18.2).

Table 18.2 Relation of ventricular tachycardia/fibrillation to infarct size and long-term treatment

	Related to infarct size	Long-term treatment
Early	Probably not	Not indicated
Late	Yes	Indicated

In contrast to early arrhythmias, ventricular tachycardia or fibrillation occurring more than 24–48 h after infarction is likely to recur days, weeks or even months later. Long-term anti-arrhythmic therapy such as sotalol or amiodarone should be prescribed. Most patients with late arrhythmias will have poor ventricular function and should therefore benefit from an angiotensin-converting enzyme inhibitor and beta-blockade. The role of the implantable cardiovertor defibrillator is discussed in chapter 25.

The more extensive the myocardial damage, the worse the prognosis. The incidence of late ventricular arrhythmias is related to the size of the infarct. However, ventricular arrhythmias are also an independent predictor of prognosis. That is, a patient with both extensive myocardial damage and late ventricular arrhythmias has a poorer prognosis than a patient with the same degree of myocardial damage but no arrhythmia (Table 18.2).

Frequent ventricular ectopic beats at the time of hospital discharge have been shown to indicate extensive myocardial damage and hence a poor prognosis but not an increased risk of arrhythmic death. There is no evidence that suppression of ventricular ectopic beats or non-sustained ventricular tachycardia improves prognosis. Studies have shown that class I anti-arrhythmic drugs actually worsen prognosis.

ASSESSMENT OF EFFICACY OF LONG-TERM ANTI-ARRHYTHMIC THERAPY

It is important to ensure that the treatment that is chosen is effective in preventing a recurrence of the arrhythmia. It should not be assumed that the oral preparation of a drug which, when given intravenously, had restored normal rhythm will be effective in preventing a recurrence of arrhythmia.

If the tachyarrhythmia has been frequent, then monitoring the electrocardiogram at the bedside or ambulatory electrocardiography are the best methods of assessing the efficacy of anti-arrhythmic therapy. Sometimes, where control has been difficult to achieve, it may be necessary to accept ventricular extrasystoles and even short runs of ventricular tachycardia, provided the rate during tachycardia is significantly slower than before treatment.

If the arrhythmia has been an infrequent event, then it is unlikely that ECG monitoring will reflect anti-arrhythmic control. Exercise ECG testing and electrophysiological testing may be helpful.

ACCELERATED IDIOVENTRICULAR RHYTHM

This is also referred to as idioventricular tachycardia or 'slow' ventricular tachycardia. It is benign and treatment is not necessary (Figure 18.9).

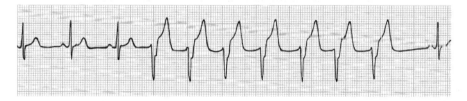

Figure 18.9 Accelerated idioventricular rhythm

SUPRAVENTRICULAR TACHYCARDIAS

AV re-entrant tachycardia can only occur if there is an additional AV connection, either bypassing or within the AV node (*see* chapter 5). Thus, it is very unlikely to occur for the first time during acute myocardial infarction. When supraventricular tachycardia is diagnosed in a patient with acute infarction, the correct diagnosis is usually atrial flutter, atrial fibrillation or even ventricular tachycardia.

ATRIAL FIBRILLATION

In atrial fibrillation, the resultant rapid ventricular rate and reduction in cardiac output from loss of atrial systole can sometimes cause severe hypotension (Figure 18.10). If shock occurs, immediate cardioversion may be necessary. Otherwise, the ventricular rate should be lowered by intravenous verapamil. If contraindicated, a beta-blocker, digoxin or amiodarone are alternatives. Spontaneous reversion to sinus rhythm is common.

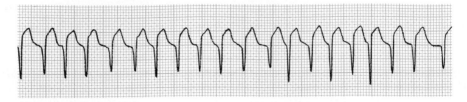

Figure 18.10 Atrial fibrillation with rapid ventricular rate in anterior infarction (lead V3)

Sustained atrial fibrillation is usually associated with extensive myocardial damage or older patients and hence a poor prognosis. Frequent atrial ectopic beats often herald atrial fibrillation.

SINUS AND JUNCTIONAL BRADYCARDIAS

Sinus and junctional bradycardias are common, particularly in inferior infarction (Figures 18.11 and 18.12). If uncomplicated, no treatment is required.

Bradycardia may be beneficial in acute infarction, in that myocardial oxygen consumption is related to heart rate and a low oxygen consumption might limit infarct size.

However, if bradycardia causes hypotension (systolic blood pressure less than 90 mmHg), mental confusion, oliguria, cold peripheries or ventricular arrhythmias,

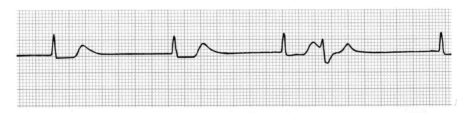

Figure 18.11 Sinus bradycardia. The fourth beat is an 'R on T' ventricular ectopic

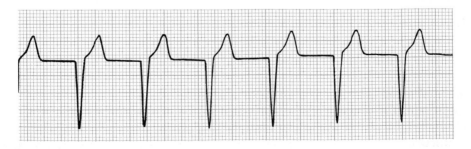

Figure 18.12 Junctional escape rhythm as a result of sinus bradycardia in anterior infarction (lead V4)

intravenous atropine (initially 0.3–0.6 mg) should be given. Temporary cardiac pacing is occasionally necessary and is preferable to frequent doses of atropine.

AV BLOCK

The management and prognosis of AV block in inferior and anterior infarction differ markedly.

INFERIOR INFARCTION

In inferior infarction, AV block is common and is often due to ischaemia of the AV node. Recovery of AV node function usually occurs within a few hours or days, although sometimes it takes up to 3 weeks. Permanent AV node damage is exceptional. The prognosis for inferior infarction is widely accepted as good, but some studies do indicate increased in-hospital mortality.

First-degree and Mobitz type I second-degree (Wenkebach) AV block require no action other than stopping drugs that may worsen AV nodal conduction, e.g. verapamil, diltiazem, beta-blockers (Figures 18.13 and 18.14).

If complete AV block develops, subsidiary pacemakers in the bundle of His will control the ventricular rate (Figure 18.15). These pacemakers usually discharge at an adequate rate. However, sometimes the ventricular rate does fall very low (less than 40 beats/min) when syncope, hypotension, mental confusion, oliguria or ventricular arrhythmia may occur. In these circumstances, temporary pacing is necessary. There is no place for steroids or catecholamines, although in the first 6 h atropine may be effective.

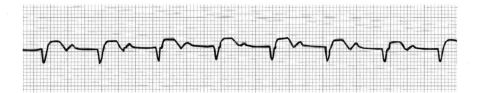

Figure 18.13 First-degree AV block (lead aVF)

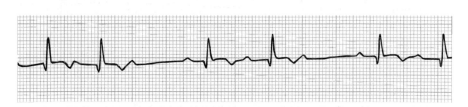

Figure 18.14 Wenkebach AV block in inferior infarction (lead aVF)

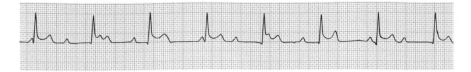

Figure 18.15 Inferior infarction complicated by complete AV block (lead II)

AV block will almost always resolve within 3 weeks of infarction, and it is highly unlikely that long-term cardiac pacing will be necessary.

ANTERIOR INFARCTION

In anterior infarction, it is the bundle branches rather than the AV node that are usually the site of ischaemic damage. AV block is more serious than in inferior infarction for two reasons. Firstly, subsidiary pacemakers that arise below the level of the block in the distal specialized conducting system tend to be slower and less reliable. Thus circulatory disturbances due to a low ventricular rate are common and ventricular standstill often occurs. Secondly, an extensive area of infarction is necessary to affect both bundle branches. Prognosis after myocardial infarction is related to the extent of infarction. Hence it is poor in patients with anterior infarction complicated by AV block.

Evidence of bilateral bundle branch damage (alternating right and left bundle branch block, or right bundle branch block with left anterior or posterior hemiblock) usually precedes the onset of second-degree (Mobitz type II) or complete AV block (Figures 18.16–18.19). The chance of bilateral bundle branch damage progressing to second-degree or complete heart block is approximately 30%. The first manifestation of these higher degrees of block may be ventricular standstill (Figure 18.20). Temporary transvenous pacing should be considered if there is evidence of bilateral bundle branch damage provided an experienced operator is available, otherwise the risks of temporary pacing will outweigh the advantages of pacing.

Second- and third-degree AV block due to anterior infarction are always indications for temporary pacing. Sinus rhythm often returns after a few days but, in some patients, AV block will persist and may necessitate long-term pacing.

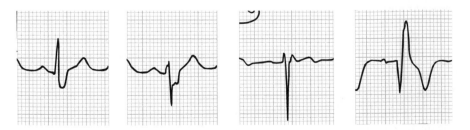

Figure 18.16 Left anterior fascicular and right bundle branch block in anterior infarction (leads I, II, III and V1)

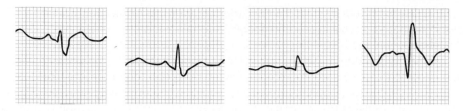

Figure 18.17 Left posterior fascicular and right bundle branch block in anterior infarction (leads I, II, III and V1)

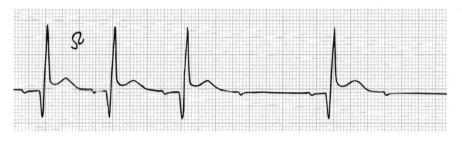

Figure 18.18 Intermittent Mobitz type II AV block in a patient with bifascicular block due to anterior infarction (lead~ V2)

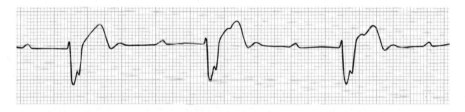

Figure 18.19 Complete AV block in anterior infarction

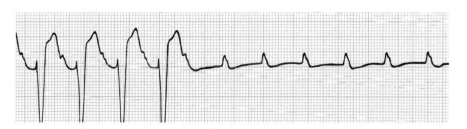

Figure 18.20 Ventricular asystole due to complete AV block in a patient with bifascicular block due to anterior infarction

Mortality is high in the first 3 weeks after anterior infarction complicated by AV block and long-term pacing should not be undertaken until the patient has survived this period.

If sinus rhythm does return, bifascicular block often persists. Complete AV block may recur in the weeks and months after acute infarction, but there is no conclusive evidence to show that implantation of a pacemaker will improve prognosis. This is because the extensive myocardial damage associated with this situation will often lead to ventricular fibrillation or heart failure.

AV DISSOCIATION

In contrast to complete AV block, the atrial rate is lower than the ventricular rate and no treatment is necessary.

Main points

- Ventricular fibrillation occurs during the first hour of acute myocardial infarction in more than 30% of patients; the incidence falls progressively thereafter.

- Frequent 'R on T' and other 'warning arrhythmias', are common in acute infarction and are not predictive of ventricular fibrillation. Anti-arrhythmic drugs are not indicated.

- Immediate defibrillation should be carried out if ventricular fibrillation occurs.

- Ventricular fibrillation or other major ventricular arrhythmia during the first 24 h of infarction is not an indication for long-term anti-arrhythmic therapy, whereas therapy should be given if these arrhythmias occur after 24 h.

- Atrial fibrillation, and ventricular arrhythmias arising 24 h or more after acute infarction, are usually associated with extensive myocardial damage and hence an impaired prognosis.

- Sinus and junctional bradycardia and complete AV block due to inferior infarction do not require treatment unless there are symptoms, marked hypotension, other signs of shock or ventricular arrhythmias. AV block due to acute inferior infarction may persist for up to 3 weeks and is not an indication for permanent pacemaker implantation.

- Bilateral bundle branch damage or higher degrees of AV block in anterior infarction imply extensive myocardial damage and a poor prognosis.

CHAPTER 19

Anti-arrhythmic drugs

LIMITATIONS

Drugs are the mainstay of treatment for arrhythmias but their limitations should be appreciated (Table 19.1).

Table 19.1 Limitations of anti-arrhythmic drugs

Limited efficacy
Unwanted effects are common
Difficulty in maintaining therapeutic drug levels
Selection of an effective drug is often based on trial and error

Anti-arrhythmic drugs are of limited effectiveness. In other words, a drug prescribed in the correct dose for an appropriate indication may fail to work.

Unwanted effects often occur. The most common are symptoms from the gastro-intestinal and central nervous systems, hypotension, heart failure and impairment of the specialized cardiac conducting tissues. Sometimes, drugs may be 'pro-arrhythmic' in that they may worsen or cause arrhythmias.

With many drugs it may be difficult to maintain consistently therapeutic drug levels.

Considerable insight into the mode of action of anti-arrhythmic drugs has been gained but selection for an individual patient of a drug that is both effective and well tolerated is often a process of trial and error.

CHOICE OF TREATMENT

Drugs are only one form of treatment and in some situations other approaches such as vagal stimulation, cardioversion, artificial pacing, catheter ablation or surgery may be more appropriate. A number of factors influence the choice of treatment: the type of arrhythmia; the urgency of the situation; the need for short- or long-term therapy; and the presence of impaired myocardial performance, sinus node dysfunction or abnormal AV conduction.

It is important to bear in mind whether an anti-arrhythmic drug is being given to terminate an arrhythmia, to prevent its recurrence or to slow the heart rate during the arrhythmia. In some situations drugs are given to control symptoms whereas in others the purpose may be to prevent dangerous arrhythmias.

PRO-ARRHYTHMIC EFFECT

Most anti-arrhythmic drugs, particularly those in class IC (see below) can worsen or cause arrhythmias, sometimes with fatal consequences. Patients with poor ventricular function are at greatest risk while the risk is very low in those with structurally normal hearts.

MODES OF ACTION

The modes of action of anti-arrhythmic drugs can be classified according to their effects in the intact heart (clinical classification) or according to their effects at cellular level as established by *in vitro* studies (action potential classification). The latter classification is widely referred to though it is of limited practical value.

CLINICAL CLASSIFICATION

Drugs are divided into three groups according to their main site or sites of action in the intact heart (Table 19.2).

Table 19.2 Classification of anti-arrhythmic actions according to principal site(s) of action in intact heart

AV node:
  Verapamil, diltiazem, adenosine, digoxin, beta-blockers

Ventricles:
  Lignocaine, mexiletine, tocainide

Atria, ventricles and accessory AV pathways:
  Quinidine, disopyramide, amiodarone, flecainide, procainamide, propafenone

The first group consists of drugs whose chief action is to slow conduction in the AV node. These drugs are therefore useful in the treatment of arrhythmias of supraventricular origin but are of little or no use in the treatment of ventricular arrhythmias. In the second group, there are drugs that work mainly in ventricular arrhythmias. The third group comprises drugs that act on the atria, ventricles and, in cases of Wolff–Parkinson–White syndrome, accessory AV pathways. Thus, they may be effective in both supraventricular and ventricular arrhythmias.

ACTION POTENTIAL CLASSIFICATION

In this classification, drugs are divided into four main classes depending upon their electrophysiological effects at cellular level (Table 19.3).

Table 19.3 Examples of action potential classification

I	II	III	IV
A. Quinidine	Beta-blockers	Amiodarone	Verapamil
Procainamide	Bretylium	Sotalol	Diltiazem
Disopyramide		Dofetilide	
		Bretylium	
Pirmenol			
B. Lignocaine			
Mexiletine			
Tocainide			
C. Flecainide			
Propafenone			
Encainide			

Class I drugs impede the transport of sodium across the cell membrane during the initiation of cellular activation and thereby reduce the rate of rise of the action potential (phase 0). Many drugs fall into this group. They are subdivided into classes A, B and C according to their effect on the duration of the action potential (which is reflected in the surface electrocardiogram by the QT interval).

IA drugs increase the duration of the action potential, IB drugs shorten it and IC drugs have little effect. The anti-arrhythmic action of IB drugs is confined to the ventricles whereas IA and IC drugs affect both atria and ventricles. IA and particularly IC drugs slow intraventricular conduction.

Class II drugs interfere with the effects of the sympathetic nervous system on the heart. They do not affect the action potential of most myocardial cells but do reduce the slope of spontaneous depolarisation (phase 4) of cells with pacemaker activity and thus the rate of pacemaker discharge.

Class III drugs prolong the duration of the action potential and hence the length of the refractory period, but do not slow phase 0.

Class IV drugs antagonize the transport of calcium across the cell membrane which follows the inward flux of sodium during cellular activation. Cells in the AV and sinus nodes are particularly susceptible. It should be noted that some calcium antagonists, e.g. nifedipine, do not have an anti-arrhythmic action.

Table 19.3 shows that the majority of drugs are in class I; drugs within this class differ significantly in their clinical effects. Some drugs have more than one class of action: amiodarone has class I, II and IV actions as well as its main class III effect! Furthermore, some drugs, e.g. digoxin and adenosine cannot be classified.

NOTES ON INDIVIDUAL DRUGS

LIGNOCAINE

Lignocaine is the first-line drug for ventricular arrhythmias but is ineffective in supraventricular arrhythmias. The drug is a vasoconstrictor and, unlike many drugs, rarely causes hypotension or heart failure.

A 100 mg bolus given intravenously over 2 min will often be successful. If not, a further bolus (50–75 mg) should be given after 5 min.

Several concentrations of lignocaine are available. Disasters have occurred because the wrong concentration has been used. Remember that 10 ml 1% lignocaine contains 100 mg.

Lignocaine is often used for short-term prevention of ventricular arrhythmias. The therapeutic effect of lignocaine is closely related to plasma levels, which fall rapidly after a bolus injection. Thus it is necessary to give a continuous infusion immediately after the bolus. There is, however, no point in giving a continuous infusion if the bolus has failed to work or, since lignocaine cannot be administered by mouth, if long-term prophylaxis is required.

It can be difficult to maintain therapeutic levels of lignocaine. With sub-therapeutic levels, the patient is at risk from arrhythmias while toxic levels may cause symptoms related to the central nervous system, including light-headedness, confusion, twitching, paraesthesiae and epileptic fits. With conventional infusion rates (1–4 mg/min) sub-therapeutic levels commonly occur in the first hour or two after the infusion is commenced.

Lignocaine is metabolized by the liver, and where there is liver disease or where hepatic blood flow is reduced by heart failure or by shock, dosages should be halved to avoid toxicity. Hypokalaemia may impair lignocaine's efficacy.

MEXILETINE

Mexiletine is similar to lignocaine in its therapeutic and haemodynamic actions, but it can be given by mouth as well as parenterally. There is a narrow margin between therapeutic and toxic effects, and symptoms such as nausea, vomiting, confusion, tremor, ataxia, as well as bradycardia and hypotension, are not uncommon.

Intravenously, the drug is given in a dose of 100–250 mg over 5–10 min, followed by 250 mg over 1 h and a further 250 mg over 2 h. The infusion can then be continued at 0.5–1.0 mg/min or oral therapy started. The oral dose is 200–300 mg 8-hourly. If the patient has not received a prior infusion, a loading dose of 400 mg can be given. Up to one-third of patients experience unwanted effects with long-term administration.The drug is mainly metabolized by the liver and doses should be reduced if there is hepatic disease or heart failure. Approximately 10% is excreted unchanged in the urine. Renal excretion is inhibited by alkaline urine but this is not a problem in practice. Though in the same anti-arrhythmic class as lignocaine, mexiletine may sometimes be effective when lignocaine has failed.

The author no longer uses this drug and does not recall the oral preparation ever having been effective!

TOCAINIDE

Tocainide is also similar to lignocaine and like mexiletine it is effective both intravenously and by mouth. Its duration of action is somewhat longer than mexiletine, making twice-daily oral administration possible. Forty per cent of the drug is excreted by the kidneys and dosage should be reduced if there is renal impairment.The intravenous dosage is 750 mg over 15 min. The daily oral dosage is 1200 mg. Side-effects include tremor, light-headedness, confusion and convulsions. There have been reports of tocainide causing agranulocytosis and thrombocytopenia. In the United Kingdom it is now recommended that the drug is only used for life-threatening ventricular arrhythmias where other drugs are ineffective or are contraindicated.

QUINIDINE

Quinidine can cause torsade de pointes tachycardia. Several surveys have shown that it increases mortality, even in patients with non-dangerous arrhythmias. The drug should not be used.

DISOPYRAMIDE

Disopyramide has been widely used for both supraventricular and ventricular arrhythmias. However, it is only moderately effective and does have significant unwanted effects.

The intravenous dose is 1.5–2.0 mg/kg up to a maximum of 150 mg, given over no less than 5 min. The injection should be stopped if the arrhythmia is terminated. Therapy can be continued by intravenous infusion at 20–30 mg/h up to a maximum of 800 mg daily or the patient can be transferred to oral therapy. The oral dose is 300–800 mg daily in three or four divided doses. If necessary a loading dose of 300 mg can be given.

Given intravenously, the drug is more likely to cause hypotension and heart failure than lignocaine and related drugs, and its use can be disastrous if the recommended minimum period of administration is ignored.

Orally, the drug's side-effects are mainly related to its anticholinergic (atropine-like) action which often causes a dry mouth, blurred vision, urinary hesitancy or retention and, by enhancing AV nodal conduction, an increase in the ventricular response to atrial flutter and fibrillation. The drug may precipitate heart failure in patients with impaired myocardial function. It may occasionally induce torsade de pointes tachycardia and should not be given to patients with QT interval prolongation. Disopyramide may worsen impaired sinus node function and is contraindicated in the sick sinus syndrome. The drug is partially excreted by the kidneys and dosage should be reduced in renal disease.

PROCAINAMIDE

Procainamide has similar anti-arrhythmic properties to quinidine. It is not widely used and, now, never by the author. It has a short half-life necessitating very frequent dosage when given by mouth. Even with a slow-release preparation, 8-hourly administration is necessary. Furthermore, unwanted effects such as systemic lupus syndrome, gastrointestinal symptoms, hypotension and agranulocytosis make it unsuitable for long-term use. Impaired renal function and a slow acetylator status both reduce procainamide requirements. N-Acetyl-procainamide, a metabolite of procainamide, has been shown to have a longer duration of action and not to cause systemic lupus.

FLECAINIDE

Flecainide is a potent drug which can be given both orally and parenterally. Its indications include ventricular arrhythmias and pre-excitation syndromes. It is very effective at suppressing ventricular ectopic beats but somewhat less so in the treatment of ventricular tachycardia.

It has a long half-life of approximately 16 h which facilitates twice daily oral administration. The dosage is 100 mg twice daily. The intravenous dose is

1–2 mg/kg body weight over not less than 10 min; it should be given more slowly in patients with impaired ventricular function. Flecainide is both metabolized by the liver and excreted by the kidney.

The drug has a narrow therapeutic range, i.e. it can be difficult to achieve a therapeutic action without unwanted effects. The most common side-effect is visual disturbance, particularly on rotating the head. Light-headedness and nausea can also occur. The drug has been shown to increase the endocardial pacing threshold.

The drug does have an important negative inotropic action and should be avoided in patients in heart failure or with extensive myocardial damage. It can be pro-arrhythmic, particularly in patients with a history of sustained ventricular tachycardia and/or poor ventricular function. In a study of patients with ventricular extrasystoles following myocardial infarction, flecainide was found to increase mortality.

Flecainide causes slight prolongation of the QRS complex and hence the QT interval; it does not prolong the JT component of the QT interval as does quinidine and disopyramide.

Flecainide is effective and safe when used to prevent atrial fibrillation and atrio-ventricular re-entrant tachycardias in patients with structurally normal hearts. It is also indicated in patients with highly symptomatic idiopathic ventricular extra-sytoles. It should be avoided in patients with myocardial damage.

Occasionally, like other class I drugs, it can worsen atrial arrhythmias: either converting atrial fibrillation to flutter, or increasing the ventricular rate during atrial flutter (Figure 19.1).

PROPAFENONE

This drug has both IC and mild beta-blocking properties and has been shown to be effective in both supraventricular and ventricular arrhythmias. It can be pro-arrhythmic and should not be given to patients with impaired ventricular function. In the author's experience, non-cardiac unwanted effects are common

AMIODARONE

Amiodarone has several advantages over other drugs. It is highly effective in both supraventricular and ventricular rhythm disorders; even in arrhythmias refractory to other drugs there is a 70% success rate. It has a remarkably long half-life (20–100 days), so that the drug need only be given once daily or even less frequently. It does not significantly impair ventricular performance and can be given to patients in heart failure.

However, it has important unwanted effects which dictate the long-term use of amiodarone being confined to patients with arrhythmias that are dangerous or resistant to other drugs, or where the risk of side-effects is not a major consideration because the patient's prognosis is poor, e.g. the elderly and those with severe myocardial damage.

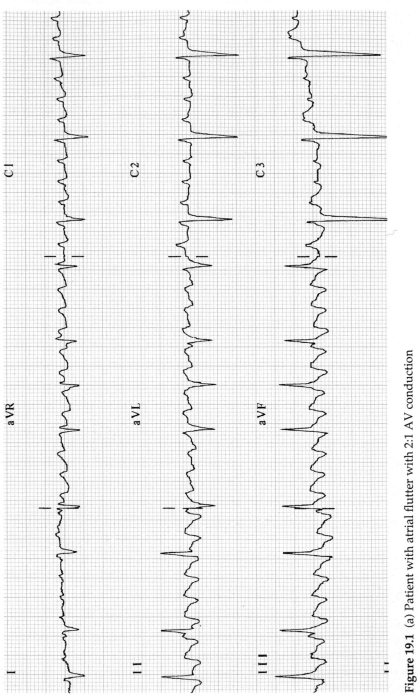

Figure 19.1 (a) Patient with atrial flutter with 2:1 AV conduction

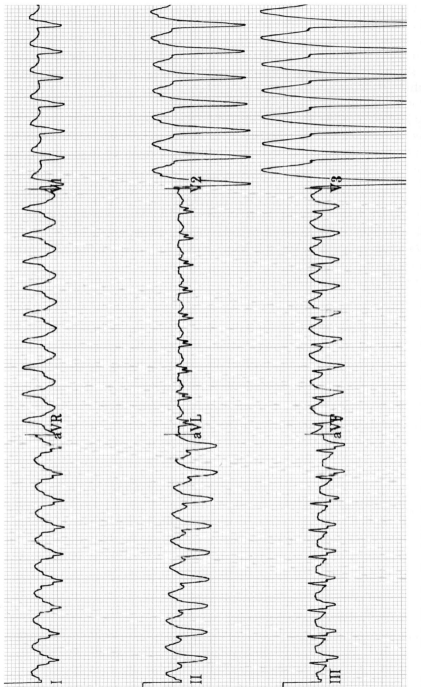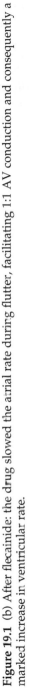

Figure 19.1 (b) After flecainide: the drug slowed the atrial rate during flutter, facilitating 1:1 AV conduction and consequently a marked increase in ventricular rate.

The drug has a delayed onset of action. When given by mouth, it usually takes 3–7 days before it takes effect and it may take 50 days to achieve its maximal action. If necessary, delay can be minimized by giving large doses, e.g. 1200 mg daily for 1 or 2 weeks. The dose can then be reduced to 400–600 mg daily.

Once the arrhythmia is controlled, it is recommended that the dose be progressively reduced until the lowest effective dose is found. The usual maintenance dose is 200–400 mg daily. In a few patients, a dose as small as 200 mg on alternate days will suffice. With dangerous arrhythmias where a recurrence cannot be risked, it is best not to reduce the dose below 400 mg daily. The drug is thought to be metabolized by the liver. It is not excreted by the kidneys. The main metabolite is desethylamiodarone which may itself have an anti-arrhythmic action. Very high concentrations of amiodarone and its metabolite are achieved in the lungs, heart, liver and adipose tissue.

Intravenous administration will lead to an earlier effect than oral therapy but, unlike most drugs, an immediate anti-arrhythmic effect does not often occur; an effect is usually seen within 1–24 h. When an arrhythmia has been difficult to control, it is often worth resorting to intravenous amiodarone in spite of possible delay in action rather than to try further drugs which are less potent and which often cause unwanted effects.

The recommended intravenous dosage is 5 mg/kg body weight over 30 min to 1 h followed by 15 mg/kg over 24 h. In an emergency, the initial infusion can be given more rapidly but its vasodilator action may cause marked hypotension. It is important to give the drug via a central venous line to avoid phlebitis. If this is not possible, frequent changes of peripheral infusion site will often suffice.

Short-term treatment with intravenous amiodarone is unlikely to cause side-effects, although a few cases of hepatitis associated with the drug have been described.

Longer term oral therapy is associated with a high incidence of side-effects. The most common are corneal microdeposits and skin photosensitivity.

Corneal microdeposits occur in virtually all patients but permanent damage does not occur. The microdeposits disappear if the drug is stopped and are a useful sign of compliance. Recently, there have been a few reports of a possible association between the drug and optic neuropathy.

Skin photosensitivity to UVA radiation affects two thirds of patients. Though only a minority experience severe photosensitivity, all patients should be warned about the possibility. If necessary, protective clothing, avoidance of prolonged sunlight and barrier creams containing zinc oxide may be recommended. Severe photosensitivity is the commonest reason for stopping the drug. A degree of photosensitivity may persist for over a year afterwards. There appears to be no relation between skin type or dosage and this unwanted effect.

After prolonged usage a minority develop marked blue–grey pigmentation of the skin: particularly the nose and forehead.

Amiodarone contains large amounts of iodine and causes elevation of both serum thyroxine and reversed tri-iodothyronine, and depression of serum tri-iodothyronine. Thyroid stimulating hormone (TSH) can be depressed. These changes are compatible with the euthyroid state. However, amiodarone can cause both hypothyroidism and hyperthyroidism. Up to 15% of patients can be affected.

Hyperthyroidism can result from activation of pre-existing subclincal thyroid disease which results in increased thyroid hormone synthesis, or from thyroiditis developing in a previously normal thyroid gland and thus increased hormone release. If hyperthyroidism occurs, the patient will often become unwell with weight loss and other signs of thyroid overactivity. Both serum thyroxine and tri-iodothyronine will be high. Amiodarone should, if possible, be stopped. Large doses of carbimazole may be required. In severe cases, short-term steroid therapy should be given. Referral to an endocrinologist is advisable. Thyroiditis may be self-limiting and there are reports of reintroduction of amiodarone without further hyperthyroidism.

If hypothyroidism occurs, serum thyroxine will be low and TSH will be elevated. Sometimes there will be no clinical signs of hypothyroidism. Thyroid hormone replacement is indicated. It is not essential to stop amiodarone.

Patients receiving long-term amiodarone should have thyroid tests at least annually.

Testicular dysfunction is another endocrine problem that may occasionally occur.

Other serious side-effects include pulmonary alveolitis, hepatitis, neuropathy and myopathy. Pulmonary alveolitis is the most common of these problems. It usually presents with dyspnoea, which may be severe, and widespread shadowing in the lung fields, which can be mistaken for pulmonary oedema. Amiodarone should be stopped and short-term therapy with steroids given. Sometimes several major unwanted effects occur together. A reduction in total diffusing capacity without clinical manifestations is common.

Usually but not invariably, serious side-effects are associated with higher dosages of amiodarone.

Other unwanted effects include nausea, rash, alopecia, tremor, insomnia and nightmares, which can be very vivid. Long-term therapy may result in a characteristic blue–grey pigmentation of the skin.

The drug's class III action results in QT prolongation, often with prominent U waves. There are a few reports of the drug causing torsade de pointes tachycardia.

It is important to note that the drug potentiates oral anticoagulants, usually halving the required dosage. Amiodarone increases blood levels of digoxin, quinidine and flecainide.

With many arrhythmias, the major advantages of amiodarone, its efficacy, absence of important negative inotropic action and long duration of action, are outweighed by the formidable list of side-effects. However, most of the side-effects are reversible and the risk of them should not be a contraindication in patients with life-threatening arrhythmias, a short life expectancy or in whom other anti-arrhythmic measures have failed.

Several studies have demonstrated that amiodarone may reduce mortality due to arrhythmias in patients with impaired ventricular function caused by myocardial infarction or cardiomyopathy but that overall or 'all cause' mortality is not influenced.

Dofetilide

Dofetilide is new class III anti-arrhyhmic drug which has been shown to be moderately successful in terminating and preventing atrial fibrillation and flutter. It does not have a negative inotropic effect.

Like amiodarone, it prolongs the QT interval. It causes torsade de pointes tachy-cardia in approximately 3% of patients. In spite of its pro-arrhythmic action, the drug was shown not to increase mortality in a large group of patients with heart failure. Torsade de pointes usually occurs within the first few days of therapy and in-hospital ECG monitoring and serial QTc measurements for at least 3 days are essential.

Orally, the usual dose is 500 mg twice daily but dosage should be reduced if there is renal impairment. If the QT interval prolongs by more than 15% after the first dose, subsequent doses should be halved. The drug should be stopped if the QTc exceeds 500 ms.

The drug should not be given to patients who have a prolonged QT interval or who are receiving verapamil, cimetidine, ketaconazole, timethoprim or pro-chlorperazine. A number of drugs including amiodarone, diltiazem, metformin, amiloride and grapefruit juice may increase blood levels.

ADENOSINE

Adenosine is a potent blocker of AV nodal conduction. It has an extremely short duration of action: 20–30 s. It is very effective in terminating supraventricular tachy-cardia due to an AV re-entrant mechanism and will transiently slow or interrupt the ventricular response to atrial fibrillation and flutter, making the respective 'f' or 'F' waves more easily identifiable. It will terminate some atrial tachycardias.

A positive response to adenosine points strongly towards a supraventricular origin to the tachycardia. However, a minority of supraventricular tachycardias will not respond to adenosine, perhaps because a dose in excess of the recommended upper limit is required, and the drug will terminate right ventricular outflow tract tachycardia. Thus, response or lack of response to adenosine is a useful pointer towards the origin of a tachycardia but cannot be taken as an absolutely reliable guide.

Adenosine was shown to be effective in terminating supraventricular tachycardia 60 years ago but it is only in the last few years that its value has been appreciated. Because of its very short duration of action and its safety, it is the drug of choice for the termination of AV and AV nodal re-entrant tachycardias.

Most patients will experience chest tightness, dyspnoea and flushing but the symptoms last less than 60 s. There may be complete AV block for a few seconds following termination of the tachycardia. The drug does not have a negative inotropic action. It is a safe drug to give except perhaps to patients with asthma in whom there is a possibility of bronchospasm. The drug is antagonized by amino-phylline and potentiated by dypiridamole. Adenosine does cause sinus bradycardia and may briefly worsen sinus node function in patients with the sick sinus syndrome.

It should be given as a rapid (2.0 s) intravenous bolus, followed by a flush of saline. The initial dose in adults and in children is 3 mg and 0.05 mg/kg, respectively. If ineffective, further dosages of 6 mg (0.10 mg/kg) and, if necessary, 12 mg (0.25 mg/kg) can be given after 1.0 min intervals.

VERAPAMIL

Intravenous verapamil (5–10 mg over 30–60 s) quickly and effectively slows AV nodal conduction. It will terminate paroxysmal (AV re-entrant) supraventricular tachycardia and will promptly slow the ventricular response to atrial fibrillation and flutter.

Orally, verapamil is less effective and because much of each dose is metabolized by the liver, large doses (40–120 mg t.d.s.) are required.

Verapamil by mouth is rarely useful alone but is very useful in combination with digoxin in controlling the ventricular response to atrial fibrillation if this cannot be achieved by apparently adequate doses of digoxin alone. Serum digoxin levels are in fact elevated by moderately large doses of verapamil.

The drug may be effective in two forms of ventricular tachycardia: right ventricular outflow tract tachycardia and fascicular tachycardia.

Intravenous verapamil is contraindicated if the patient has received an intravenous or oral beta-blocker. Profound bradycardia or hypotension can result and may be fatal. Sometimes, the combination of oral verapamil and a beta-blocker will cause profound sinus or junctional bradycardia. Verapamil is contraindicated in patients with impaired sinus or AV node function or digoxin toxicity unless a ventricular pacing wire is *in situ* because of its depressant effects on the sinus and AV nodes.

Verapamil does have a significant negative inotropic effect and may cause hypotension in patients with very poor myocardial function. Two studies report that administration of intravenous calcium chloride immediately prior to parenteral verapamil prevents hypotension.

BETA-ADRENOCEPTOR ANTAGONISTS

These drugs have anti-arrhythmic properties by virtue of their principal action: antagonizing the effects of catecholamines on the heart. They are most effective in arrhythmias caused by increased sympathetic nervous system activity, e.g. those caused by exertion, emotion, thyrotoxicosis, acute myocardial infarction and the hereditary QT prolongation syndromes.

Beta-blocking drugs slow AV nodal conduction and thus, like verapamil, are useful in arrhythmias of supraventricular origin. Unwanted bradycardia caused by beta-blockade can usually be quickly reversed by atropine.

Intravenous esmolol has an extremely short half-life of only 2 min. Its beta-adrenoceptor antagonist action and any associated unwanted effects will therefore be brief.

SOTALOL

Sotalol, in addition to its beta-blocking property, prolongs the duration of the action potential and hence QT interval; it has a significant class III, or amiodarone-like action. Unlike other beta-blockers, sotalol has a marked effect upon the recovery periods of atrial and ventricular myocardium and accessory AV pathways.

It has a long half-life and can be given once daily. The oral dosage is 160–240 mg daily. The drug is excreted by the kidneys: dosage should be reduced if renal function is impaired. Intravenously, it should be given slowly up to a dosage of 1.5 mg/kg.

There are reports of the drug – usually in association with other drugs or hypokalaemia – of causing torsade de pointes tachycardia.

Sotalol is considerably more effective than other beta-blockers for prevention of atrial fibrillation and other supraventricular arrhythmias, and also has an important role in the treatment of ventricular arrhythmias.

For many arrhythmias, it should be considered a first-line drug though, of course, it cannot be used in cases when beta-blockers are contraindicated.

DIGOXIN

The main use of digoxin is as an AV nodal blocking drug in the control of the ventricular rate during atrial fibrillation. The usual dose is 0.25–0.375 mg daily. A number of factors – e.g. hypokalaemia, renal impairment, dehydration (often caused by diuretics) and therapy with quinidine, verapamil or amiodarone – predispose to digoxin toxicity and are an indication for dosage reduction.

Digoxin toxicity

Digoxin toxicity is a common problem. Over 10% of patients receiving the drug who are admitted to hospital have been found to have evidence of digoxin toxicity.

A number of symptoms suggest digoxin toxicity. These include anorexia, nausea, vomiting, diarrhoea, mental confusion, xanthopsia and visual blurring. However, none of these symptoms is specific to digoxin toxicity; in patients with severe congestive heart failure, in particular, gastrointestinal symptoms are often caused by heart failure rather than digoxin.

Digoxin toxicity can cause a number of disorders of cardiac rhythm. These include atrial tachycardia with AV block (Figure 19.2), junctional tachycardia (Figure 19.3), ventricular ectopic beats (often bigeminy) (Figure 19.4), ventricular tachycardia, first-, second- and third-degree AV block, a slow ventricular response to atrial fibrillation (Figure 19.5) and sino-atrial block (Figure 19.6).

The main use of digoxin is to control the ventricular rate during atrial fibrillation. When a patient receiving digoxin for this purpose develops a regular pulse, a

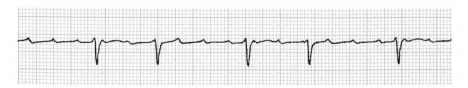

Figure 19.2 Atrial tachycardia with varying degrees of AV block

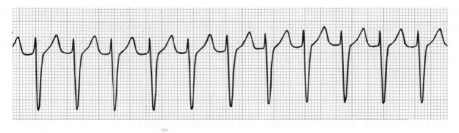

Figure 19.3 Junctional tachycardia

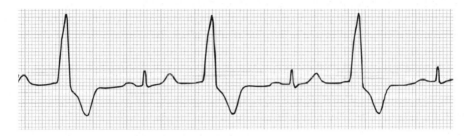

Figure 19.4 First-degree AV block with ventricular bigeminy

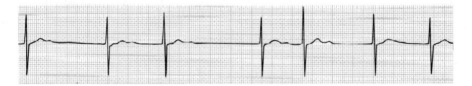

Figure 19.5 Slow ventricular response to atrial fibrillation

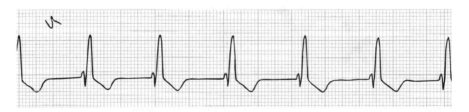

Figure 19.6 Junctional rhythm

number of possibilities should be considered. First, sinus rhythm may have returned. Secondly, an arrhythmia due to digoxin toxicity may have developed, e.g. atrial tachycardia with AV block, junctional tachycardia or atrial fibrillation with complete AV block. Without an ECG it may be difficult to ascertain whether the regular rhythm is due to an arrhythmia or not.

Plasma digoxin levels can be measured but must be interpreted in conjunction with clinical features. Levels less than 1.5 ng/ml, in the absence of hypokalaemia, indicate that digoxin toxicity is unlikely. Levels in excess of 3.0 ng/ml indicate that toxicity is probable. With levels between 1.5 and 3.0 ng/ml digoxin toxicity should be considered a possibility, particularly if there are symptoms or arrhythmias attributable to digoxin toxicity or if there is renal impairment, or if the patient appears to be on an inappropriately large dose of digoxin. Blood for digoxin concentration estimation must be taken at least 6 h after the last dose.

Usually temporary discontinuation of the drug and correction of hypokalaemia, if present, are all that is required. Serious ventricular arrhythmias should be treated with intravenous anti-arrhythmic drugs. Lignocaine is suitable, though animal studies suggest that Epanutin (phenytoin) may be preferable. It has also been suggested that beta-blockers are particularly effective; these, however, may worsen AV node function and increase the risk of AV block developing. Specific digoxin-binding antibodies can be used in serious cases of toxicity.

If high degrees of AV block occur, temporary cardiac pacing may be necessary. Cardioversion is dangerous in the presence of digoxin toxicity. If cardioversion is essential, low energy levels, e.g. 5–10 J, increasing gradually as necessary, should be used and lignocaine 75–100 mg should be given.

ANTI-ARRHYTHMIC DRUGS DURING PREGNANCY

No anti-arrhythmic drug is completely safe during pregnancy. Where possible, drugs should be avoided in patients with well-tolerated arrhythmias, particularly in the first trimester.

Of the commonly used drugs, beta-blockers and flecainide have been used quite widely and appear relatively safe. Amiodarone has been reported to cause congenital abnormalities.

THERAPEUTIC RANGE OF PLASMA LEVELS

The therapeutic range of plasma levels of the commonly used anti-arrhythmic drugs are given in Table 19.4. However, measurement of plasma levels is of limited use and is not often necessary in routine treatment.

If there is good evidence of a therapeutic effect with a standard dosage regimen and there are no unwanted effects, measurement of a drug's plasma level is of little importance. However, knowledge of a drug's level may be helpful with some clinical problems, e.g. when there is doubt as to whether a patient is taking his or her therapy or as to whether symptoms may be due to drug toxicity.

Table 19.4 Therapeutic range of plasma levels (µg/ml) for some anti-arrhythmic drugs

Amiodarone	1.0–2.5
Disopyramide	2.0–6.0
Flecainide	0.2–1.0
Lignocaine	1.4–6.0
Mexiletine	0.5–2.0
Procainamide	4.0–10.0
Quinidine	2.3–5.0
Tocainide	6.0–12.0
Verapamil	100–200

Main points

- Anti-arrhythmic drugs are of limited efficacy and often cause unwanted effects.

- Choice of anti-arrhythmic therapy should be tailored to the individual patient and depends on the arrhythmia, the degree of associated circulatory disturbance, the presence of impaired myocardial, sinus node or AV node function, need for short- or long-term treatment and concurrent administration of other drugs.

- Drugs are usually better at terminating arrhythmias than at preventing their recurrence.

- Disopyramide, flecainide and beta-blockers have a marked negative inotropic action and may precipitate heart failure in patients with extensive myocardial damage.

- Many drugs can have a pro-arrhythmic action, particularly if ventricular function is impaired.

- Adenosine is the treatment of choice for termination of AV re-entrant tachycardias.

- Intravenous verapamil will quickly control the ventricular response to atrial fibrillation and flutter. It should not be given to a patient who has received a beta-blocker.

- Lignocaine is the first-line drug for termination of ventricular tachycardia.

- Sotalol is effective in a wide variety of arrhythmias.

- Amiodarone is the most effective anti-arrhythmic agent currently available, but its long-term use should be confined to the treatment of patients with arrhythmias that are dangerous or are refractory to other forms of treatment, or who have a poor prognosis.

Cardioversion

Electrical cardioversion is the use of an electric shock of brief duration and high energy to terminate a tachyarrhythmia. The shock depolarizes the myocardium, thus interrupting the tachycardia and allowing the sinus node to resume control of the heart rhythm.

Chemical cardioversion is the restoration of normal rhythm by anti-arrhythmic drugs and is discussed elesewhere.

TRANSTHORACIC CARDIOVERSION

Cardioversion is usually carried out by delivering a shock between two electrodes placed on the chest.

PROCEDURE

Facilities for monitoring the ECG and for cardiopulmonary resuscitation must be available.

The rhythm should be checked immediately before cardioversion to ensure that spontaneous reversion has not occurred.

Anaesthesia

A conscious patient should receive a short-acting anaesthetic, or an intravenous amnesic agent, e.g. midazolam or diazepam. The patient should fast for 4 h before elective cardioversion.

Delivery of shock

The shock is delivered with two electrode paddles. Correct positioning is essential. Usually one electrode is placed at the level of the cardiac apex, close to the mid-axillary line, and the other is positioned to the right of the upper sternum.

Alternatively, a flat paddle, if available, can be placed beneath the patient's back, behind the heart, and a second paddle positioned over the praecordium. Standard paddles can be applied anteroposteriorly if the patient is turned on to his or her side; one paddle is placed over the praecordium and the other paddle below the left shoulder to the left of the spine.

To achieve good electrical contact and to avoid burning the skin, electrode jelly must be applied to the areas beneath the paddles. However, it is essential to avoid spreading jelly between the two paddles. Pads impregnated with electrode gel prevent jelly being spread over inappropriate areas, including the operator!

The cardiovertor is charged to the desired energy level (see below), which takes a few seconds. The charge is usually released by pressing the button(s) on the defibrillator paddle(s). Application of the paddles with firm pressure reduces the electrical resistance of the thorax.

Before discharge it is essential to ensure that no one is in contact with the patient.

If cardioversion is unsuccessful, depending on the circumstances, further shocks with higher energy levels may be tried.

The heart rhythm should be monitored after cardioversion.

Synchronization

Ventricular fibrillation may be induced if a shock coincides with the ventricular T wave. Therefore, defibrillators have a mechanism whereby discharge is triggered to occur on the R or S wave. This mechanism should be used during cardioversion for all arrhythmias except ventricular fibrillation. With ventricular fibrillation, there will be no detectable R wave and, thus, if the mechanism is in operation, the defibrillator will not discharge.

Before synchronized cardioversion, the operator should check that the synchronizing signal coincides with the onset of the QRS complex. Sometimes, the amplitude of the ECG has to be increased to enable synchronization.

Energy levels

In general, low energy levels are used initially. If unsuccessful, further shocks can be given at increased levels. For most arrhythmias, the initial level should be 100 J, increasing by 100 J steps to 300 J if necessary.

Atrial flutter usually responds to low-energy shocks; 50 J is a suitable initial level. On the other hand, with ventricular fibrillation the initial energy should be 200 J.

When digoxin toxicity is likely, very low levels should be used, starting at 5–10 J.

Complications

Complications are rare.

Cardioversion often causes marked elevation in creatinine kinase but does not elevate troponin levels. Thus, cardioversion may affect skeletal muscle but does not cause myocardial damage.

Transient arrhythmias occasionally occur but these are rarely a problem unless there is digoxin toxicity.

In patients with the bradycardia–tachycardia syndrome cardioversion may cause a major bradycardia; a temporary pacing wire should be inserted before cardioversion.

Systemic embolism may occur when cardioversion is carried out for atrial fibrillation (see below).

DIGOXIN TOXICITY

Cardioversion in digoxin toxicity can produce dangerous ventricular arrhythmias. For this reason, cardioversion should be a last resort and should be preceded by lignocaine 75–100 mg.

Because of the dangers of digoxin toxicity, it has become common practice to stop digoxin for 24–48 h before cardioversion. However, cardioversion in the presence of therapeutic levels of digoxin is safe. There is no need to postpone cardioversion if the patient is receiving standard doses of digoxin, renal function and plasma electrolytes are normal, and there are no symptoms or ECG findings suggestive of digoxin toxicity (*see* chapter 19).

Implanted pacemaker

Cardioversion may cause pacemaker damage unless the paddles are at least 15 cm from the generator and preferably are positioned so they are at right angles to the line between the pacemaker generator and the heart. Pacemaker function should be checked after the procedure.

INDICATIONS

Ventricular fibrillation

Immediate cardioversion is necessary. The initial energy level should be 200 J. If unsuccessful, a further 200 J shock should be given. If ventricular fibrillation persists, a 360 J shock should be delivered (*see* chapter 21).

Recent developments in defibrillation include the use of biphasic rather than sinusoidal waveforms, and automated defibrillators.

Sequential or simultaneous shocks, delivered by means of two defibrillators with separate pairs of electrodes, should be considered in any patient who does not defibrillate with repeated 360-J shocks.

Ventricular tachycardia

Cardioversion is indicated if the arrhythmia causes shock or cardiac arrest, or if drug therapy has failed. With very fast ventricular tachycardias it may be difficult to synchronize delivery of the shock and it may be necessary to deliver an unsychronized shock.

Atrial fibrillation

Sinus rhythm can be restored by cardioversion in most patients with atrial fibrillation. However, not infrequently the arrhythmia returns.

High-energy shocks are often required. 200 J should be used for the first shock. A shock of 360 J applied between anterior and posterior paddles is often successful in resistant cases, and cardioversion should not be deemed to be unsuccessful unless this has been tried.

ANTICOAGULATION

Cardioversion of atrial fibrillation can result in systemic embolism because of dislodgement of pre-existing thrombus. New atrial thrombus can develop after cardioversion because atrial mechanical activity often does not return for up to 3 weeks after the procedure. Hence embolism can also occur in the following few weeks. It is therefore recommended that nonurgent cardioversion in patients who have been in atrial fibrillation for more than 24 h is preceded by warfarin for at least 3 weeks, and is continued for at least 4 weeks after restoration of normal rhythm.

If warfarin is not given prior to cardioversion because it has to be carried out urgently or because the arrhythmia had persisted for less than 48 h, the procedure should be preceded by intravenous heparin.

While cardioversion only leads to long-term sinus rhythm in a minority of patients, an attempt at restoring sinus rhythm should be considered in those patients with recent atrial fibrillation (less than 12 months) where no cause has been identified or in whom the disorder which has caused the arrhythmia has resolved or is self-limiting. Cardioversion should be considered in those patients with atrial fibrillation which has been present for more than 12 months, if symptoms due to the arrhythmia are severe even there is only a small chance of long-term normal rhythm.

If there is a recurrence, a further attempt at cardioversion, after initiation of antiarrhythmic therapy, should only be undertaken in those with troublesome symptoms attributable to the arrhythmia. Several drugs such as disopyramide, flecainide, sotalol and, especially, amiodarone reduce the relapse rate after cardioversion.

Atrial flutter

This arrhythmia, which is often difficult to treat with drugs, responds to low-energy shocks. The need for anticoagulation is controversial. The risk of embolism is lower than with atrial fibrillation. However, flutter and fibrillation can sometimes coexist, so some recommend the same anticoagulant regime as for atrial fibrillation. Anticoagulation is definitely indicated if there is myocardial or valve disease, or a history of embolism.

Though cardioversion is almost always successful, atrial flutter will recur in half of cases.

AV re-entrant tachycardia

Cardioversion is indicated on the few occasions when other measures, such as vagal stimulation or intravenous adenosine, or verapamil, have failed.

TRANSVENOUS CARDIOVERSION

Recently, transvenous cardioversion has been introduced. A low-energy shock is delivered between transvenous electrodes positioned in the right atrium and either the coronary sinus or left pulmonary artery. A single-lead, balloon-guided system is now available which also facilitates atrial and ventricular pacing, if required.

Higher success rates than for transthoracic cardioversion have been reported, especially in very large patients.

Main points

- The usual positions for the defibrillator paddles are the cardiac apex and to the right of the upper sternum.

- Firm paddle pressure should be applied prior to delivery of the DC shock.

- Except for ventricular fibrillation, delivery of the shock should be synchronized to the R or S wave of the electrocardiogram.

- Initial energy levels depend on the clinical circumstances: 50 J for atrial flutter, 200 J for ventricular fibrillation, 100 J for most other arrhythmias. 300 J is often required to cardiovert atrial fibrillation.

- Digoxin toxicity is a contraindication to cardioversion.

- Temporary transvenous pacing should precede cardioversion if the brady-cardia–tachycardia syndrome is suspected.

- In patients with atrial fibrillation or flutter due to conditions associated with a significant risk from systemic embolism, oral anticoagulation should precede cardioversion.

- Damage to an implanted pacemaker or defibrillator can be prevented if the paddles are placed at least 15 cm from the generator and preferably positioned so they are at right angles to the pacing system.

Cardiopulmonary resuscitation

Cardiac arrest is the cessation of an effective cardiac output as the result of a sudden circulatory or respiratory catastrophe. Patients dying of terminal and irreversible diseases will not benefit from and should not undergo the indignity of cardiopulmonary resuscitation.

COMMON CAUSES OF CARDIAC ARREST

1. Acute myocardial infarction.
2. Severe coronary artery disease.
3. Myocardial damage resulting from past infarction, cardiomyopathy or myocarditis.
4. Anoxia, e.g. due to drowning, smoke inhalation, airways obstruction, or respiratory depression.
5. Electrocution.
6. Iatrogenic, e.g. hypokalaemia, or overdose of opiate or catecholamine.
7. Anaphylactic response to a drug or other allergen.

CARDIOPULMONARY RESUSCITATION

Management of cardiac arrest consists of three stages:

1. basic life support;
2. advanced life support;
3. aftercare.

Speed and efficiency in the diagnosis and management of cardiac arrest are crucial. The shorter the delays in starting basic life support and in restoring normal heart action, the more likely is a successful outcome. Resuscitation of adults is discussed below.

Basic life support

This term refers to the combination of external chest compression and expired air respiration. Equipment and drugs are not required. The purpose of basic life support is to maintain adequate ventilation and circulation until means can be obtained to reverse the underlying cause of the arrest. Occasionally, particularly when arrest has been due to respiratory failure, it may itself reverse the cause and allow full recovery.

Diagnosis of cardiac arrest is based on three signs:

1. unconsciousness;
2. cessation of breathing;
3. absent carotid or femoral artery pulsation.

Expired air respiration

With the palm of one hand, tilt the patient's head backwards so that the neck is fully extended. With the fingers of the other hand, lift the lower jaw forward so that it protrudes beyond the upper teeth. Without these manoeuvres the tongue will obstruct the airway and artificial ventilation will be impossible.

Mouth-to-mouth respiration should then be given by taking a deep breath and, after pinching the patient's nose and sealing the lips around those of the patient, blowing forcefully into the patient's mouth for 1.5–2.0 s. The patient's chest should be seen to rise, otherwise ventilation is inadequate. If chest expansion is not achieved, the pharynx should be examined to ensure that it is not obstructed by vomit or foreign material.

External chest compression

The heel of one hand is placed over the sternum at the junction of its upper two-thirds and lower one-third and is covered by the other hand. Keeping the arms straight, and with the shoulders directly aligned above the hands, the sternum should be depressed 4–5 cm at a rate of 100 beats/min. Each compression should be sustained so that the time spent in compression is equal to that of relaxation.

If there is only one rescuer, after each 15 compressions, there should be a pause to deliver two expired air inflations. If there are two rescuers, after each five compressions there should be a pause for one expired air inflation.

Mechanism
Chest compression was thought to work by squeezing the ventricles between the sternum and vertebrae thereby expelling blood into the arteries. Hence the older

term 'cardiac massage'. However, it is now known that chest compression increases intrathoracic pressure and thereby propels blood into the systemic arteries. Valves at the superior thoracic inlet prevent regurgitation into the venous system and, between chest compressions, the aortic valve remains competent, thus preventing blood flowing back into the heart.

One piece of evidence that supports that the heart is a passive conduit during chest compression may be of practical value: rapid, vigorous coughing at the onset of ventricular fibrillation may generate sufficient cardiac output to maintain consciousness.

Optimal chest compression only achieves one-third of normal cardiac output.

ADVANCED LIFE SUPPORT

Treatment depends on the heart rhythm. The paddles of a modern defibrillator also function as electrodes, enabling the heart rhythm to be quickly ascertained.

The ECG may reveal ventricular fibrillation, ventricular tachycardia, asystole or, rarely, sinus rhythm. The latter may occur as a result of electromechanical dissociation, pulmonary embolism, cardiac tamponade or tension pneumothorax.

Ventricular fibrillation

Occasionally, a single blow to the praecordium with the side of a clenched first will, if given shortly after the onset of ventricular fibrillation (or tachycardia), restore sinus rhythm. Otherwise, the patient should be immediately defibrillated. Time should not be wasted with basic life support procedures if a defibrillator is to hand. To avoid one common cause of delay, it is essential to ensure familiarity with the controls of the available defibrillator(s).

The defibrillator should be charged to 200 J. One paddle should be firmly applied to the right of the upper sternum and the other to the cardiac apex after having placed electrode jelly or pads impregnated with electrode gel beneath the paddles. Everyone should be instructed to avoid contact with the patient who is then defibrillated by depressing the button(s) on the defibrillator paddle(s).

In patients with implanted pacemakers or defibrillators, a paddle should not be positioned within 15 cm of the device.

If ventricular fibrillation persists, a further 200 J shock should be given. The majority of episodes of ventricular fibrillation will be terminated by the first or second 200 J shock. If the second attempt at defibrillation is unsuccessful a shock of 360 J should be given. Further action for persistent ventricular fibrillation is detailed in the summary below (i.e. step 4 and onwards).

Sequential shocks, delivered by means of two defibrillators with separate pairs of electrodes, should be considered in any patient who does not defibrillate with repeated 360-J shocks.

Endotracheal intubation should not be carried out unless first attempts at restoring normal heart action (see below) are unsuccessful.

Nitrate patches or paste should be removed from the chest.

SUMMARY OF SEQUENCE OF ACTIONS FROM ONSET OF VENTRICULAR FIBRILLATION

1. 200 J shock
2. 200 J shock
3. 360 J shock

4. endotracheal intubation
5. insertion of venous cannula

6. adrenaline 1 mg (i.e. 10 mls 1:10000 soln)
7. chest compression and ventilation – 10 sequences
8. 360 J shock
9. 360 J shock
10. 360 J shock

11. repeat steps 6–10, three times
12. consider i.v. amiodarone or lignocaine
13. change paddle positions, e.g. axilla to axilla, or anteroposterior.

The purpose of adrenaline is to increase peripheral resistance and thereby divert blood flow to the myocardium. Experiments in animals suggest that this facilitates defibrillation though recent observations in man suggest that adrenaline may possibly have a deleterious effect. Sodium bicarbonate used to be given in large doses at the start of cardiopulmonary resuscitation to reverse acidosis, but it is now appreciated that this practice is not necessary and may be harmful.

Ventricular tachycardia

When ventricular tachycardia causes cardiac arrest, it is preferable to set the synchronizing mechanism so that the shock falls on the R wave rather than the T wave to avoid the risk of inducing ventricular fibrillation. Remember, if the synchronization button is depressed, it will not be possible to deliver a shock during ventricular fibrillation since no R waves will be detected.

Asystole

Resuscitation from asystole is often successful when the cause is anoxia or disease confined to the specialized conducting tissues. In the former case ventilation may be all that is required. In the latter case the mechanical stimulation of repeated praecordial blows or cardiac massage may initiate ventricular activation. On the other hand, when asystole is due to extensive myocardial damage, successful resuscitation is unlikely.

Occasionally, an ECG trace during an arrest may be flat, suggesting asystole and yet the arrest is due to ventricular fibrillation: the gain on the ECG may be too low, there may be a fault in the leads or the fibrillatory waves may be of very low amplitude. If there is any doubt, ventricular fibrillation should be assumed and steps 1–3 in the above series of defibrillator discharges given.

If ventricular fibrillation has been excluded, 10 ml 1:10000 adrenaline should be given. Ten sequences of chest compression and ventilation should then be applied. If asystole persists, adrenaline and the chest compression sequence should be repeated three times.

If the patient is still asystolic, atropine 3 mg and then further adrenaline may be tried.

Occasionally ventricular standstill may occur during atrial fibrillation and be confused with fine ventricular fibrillation.

Pacing is rarely effective unless asystole is due to disease of the specialized conducting tissues.

Sinus rhythm

In patients with myocardial damage, electromechanical dissociation, i.e. persistence of electrical activity without mechanical activity can sometimes be reversed with intravenous adrenaline or 10 ml 10% calcium chloride.

If cardiac arrest is thought to be due to cardiac tamponade, immediate aspiration of the pericardium or thoracotomy is indicated. Transfusion should be given if arrest is due to severe hypovolaemia. Where pulmonary embolism is suspected, 15 000 units heparin should be given intravenously. If facilities are to hand, emergency pulmonary embolectomy may be possible.

Administration of drugs

Drugs should be given via a large vein, e.g. antecubital vein. Any drug given should be flushed through with saline. If necessary, a line can be inserted into a central vein. The femoral vein is a good approach, since it is remote from the area of resuscitation. The external jugular vein is often distended during cardiac arrest, allowing easy cannulation. In some patients it may be necessary to cannulate the internal jugular or subclavian vein.

If it is impossible to insert a venous line, adrenaline and lignocaine can be given via the intrapulmonary route. They should be diluted in 10 ml saline and be given through a fine catheter, introduced via the endotracheal tube, deep into the lungs. Doses should be double those used intravenously.

AFTERCARE

The patient should be transferred to an intensive or coronary care unit. The heart rhythm should be monitored during transfer. If the patient has not fully regained consciousness, the need for artificial ventilation should be considered.

Blood should be sent to check blood electrolytes and arterial gases. A chest X-ray should be done.

Severe acidosis (pH < 7.1) should be reversed with 50 ml 8.4% sodium bicarbonate.

OUT-OF-HOSPITAL SUDDEN CARDIAC DEATH

Sudden death due to cardiac disease is common. The annual incidence in the United Kingdom has been estimated to be in excess of 75 000. The mechanism is usually ventricular tachycardia or fibrillation. Ventricular fibrillation often results from degeneration from ventricular tachycardia rather than being the primary arrhythmia.

Coronary heart disease is by far the most common cause. Though acute myocardial infarction commonly leads to ventricular fibrillation, it accounts for less than one-third of patients presenting with sudden death. The majority have been found to have extensive coronary disease and poor left ventricular but not acute infarction. Other causes include dilated and hypertrophic cardiomyopathies, myocarditis, Wolff–Parkinson–White syndrome and hereditary prolongation of the QT interval. Sudden death due to chest wall impact during sports (Commotio cordis) has been reported. It is caused by a praecordial blow coincident with the T wave causing ventricular fibrillation.

Several centres, mainly in North America, have shown that facilities for out-of-hospital cardiopulmonary resuscitation do save lives. As a result, information on the syndrome of 'aborted sudden cardiac death' is increasing. It is now clear that patients who are resuscitated and who have not sustained acute infarction remain at risk. There is a recurrence rate of up to 60% within 2 years.

Patients resuscitated from cardiac arrest not caused by acute infarction must be investigated to assess the need for myocardial revascularization, anti-arrhythmic drug therapy or implantation of an automatic defibrillator before discharge from hospital.

Main points

- Loss of consciousness, apnoea and absence of carotid or femoral artery pulsation are the only signs required for the diagnosis of cardiac arrest.

- Chest compression is often poorly performed. Correct positioning of the hands, at the junction of the upper two-thirds and lower-third of the sternum, is essential. The operator's arms should be kept straight by 'locking the elbows', with the shoulder positioned directly above the hands. The chest should be compressed at a rate of 100 beats/min, the duration of each compression should be sustained and equal to the relaxation phase.

- Maintenance of a clear airway by full extension of the neck is essential for effective mouth-to-mouth resuscitation.

- If there is ventricular fibrillation, the sooner defibrillation is carried out the more likely a successful outcome. Initially, 200 J should be delivered, the two paddles being positioned at the cardiac apex and to the right of the upper sternum. To avoid one common cause of delay, there should be familiarity with the controls of the defibrillator(s) that one is likely to use.

- Out-of-hospital sudden cardiac death is usually due to ventricular tachy-cardia or fibrillation resulting from coronary heart disease. Frequently, there will be no evidence of acute myocardial infarction: without treatment recurrence is likely.

CHAPTER 22

Ambulatory ECG monitoring

PROLONGED ECG RECORDING

The standard resting electrogram records the heart rhythm for no more than 30 s and is, therefore, not suitable for detecting intermittent disturbances in heart rhythm. Ambulatory ECG monitoring is an invaluable diagnostic tool. The ECG can be continuously or intermittently recorded for long periods.

CONTINUOUS ECG RECORDING

The ECG can be continuously recorded, usually for 24–48 h, using a portable battery-operated recorder, which is usually worn on a belt at the waist. The ECG is either recorded as an analogue signal on tape, or in digital form in solid-state recording systems. If appropriate, the patient can be fully ambulant, carrying out his or her normal day-to-day activities.

The ECG is recorded by means of two electrodes applied to areas of thoroughly cleaned skin. Usually one electrode is placed over the manubrium sterni and the other electrode over the V5 chest lead position. As an alternative, a modified V1 lead can be obtained by placing one electrode over the V1 chest lead position and the other electrode beneath the lateral part of the left clavicle.

Most systems allow simultaneous recording of two leads. This increases diagnostic accuracy and aids in the detection of artefact, which is unlikely to appear on both leads at the same time (Figure 22.1). Furthermore, sometimes one lead will not reveal important diagnostic information while the other will (Figure 22.2).

The recording is analysed by replaying it at 60–100 times real-time. Playback systems have facilities for printing out selected portions of the recording on ECG paper at standard speed. Most recording systems can automatically detect brady-cardias, tachycardias and ectopic beats, though in practice an operator has to supervise the analysis.

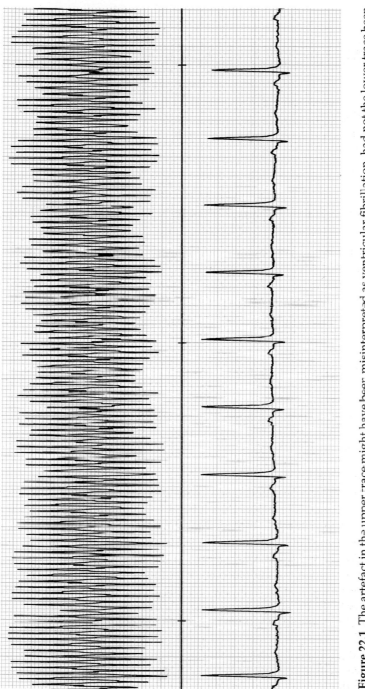

Figure 22.1 The artefact in the upper trace might have been misinterpreted as ventricular fibrillation, had not the lower trace been recorded simultaneously

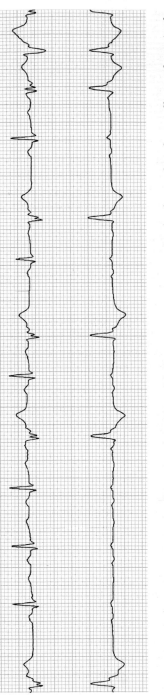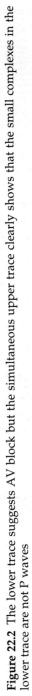

Figure 22.2 The lower trace suggests AV block but the simultaneous upper trace clearly shows that the small complexes in the lower trace are not P waves

Clinical applications

Ambulatory ECG monitoring enables the detection and diagnosis of intermittent disorders of cardiac rhythm and may thus reveal the cause of symptoms such as syncope, palpitation and chest pain.

The technique is most valuable when the patient experiences his or her usual symptoms during an ECG recording. The patient should be instructed to record the time of onset of the symptoms so these can be correlated with the heart rhythm. With some recorders the patient can operate an event marker which indicates the time of symptoms on the tape.

Even when the patient does not experience symptoms during a recording, rhythm abnormalities of diagnostic significance may be detected. Obviously, if the patient does not experience symptoms during the recording and no rhythm abnormalities are found, an arrhythmic cause for the patient's symptoms is not excluded. In the absence of typical symptoms, the finding of a minor abnormality of rhythm does not rule out a more major rhythm disturbance being responsible for the patient's complaints.

It may sometimes be necessary to record several tapes to obtain diagnostic information.

ANTI-ARRHYTHMIC THERAPY

Ambulatory monitoring is of some value in assessing a patient's response to therapy. For example, not uncommonly ambulatory electrocardiography will reveal frequent ventricular arrhythmias despite the use of an anti-arrhythmic agent. One problem in using ambulatory monitoring to assess therapy is that there is a marked spontaneous variation in the frequency of arrhythmias and so, based on one recording, absence or improvement in arrhythmia may not necessarily be a result of drug therapy.

More importantly, ambulatory electrocardiography may reveal a drug's pro-arrhythmic effect.

'Normal' findings

Sinus bradycardia, short pauses, up to 2 s, due to sino-atrial block, first-degree and AV Wenkebach block can occur in normal people during sleep and should not be regarded as evidence of conduction tissue disease. These rhythms may also occur during the day in young people with high vagal tone. Sinus tachycardia will of course also be seen in recordings from people with normal hearts.

Whereas a routine 12-lead electrocardiogram records approximately 60 heartbeats, a normal 24-h tape recording is likely to contain at least 90 000 beats. Thus ambulatory electrocardiography is a much more sensitive tool than a standard recording. For example, the finding of a single ventricular ectopic beat on a routine ECG suggests a much higher frequency than a hundred ectopic beats on a 24-h tape. In fact, studies of apparently normal people using ambulatory electrocardiography have shown that unifocal ventricular extrasystoles occur commonly, as do supraventricular ectopic beats. The frequency of ventricular ectopic beats increases with age. Some studies have also found short runs of relatively slow ventricular tachycardia in apparently normal young subjects.

Nonsustained ventricular tachycardia rarely occurs in subjects without structural heart disease and is not associated with risk.

Artefacts

Several technical problems during ambulatory electrocardiography can result in what appear to be arrhythmias to the unwary.

If the tape speed slows for any reason, complexes will appear closer together and mimic tachycardia. However, the duration of each ventricular complex will be shorter than normal and this should alert the observer to the likelihood of artefact. Conversely, if the tape runs too fast, apparent bradycardia with broader than normal complexes will result.

Not infrequently, a lead will become disconnected during a recording. Since no activity is being recorded, the ECG will appear as a straight line and mimic sinus arrest. Furthermore, sometimes an electrical connection can intermittently fail, resulting in repeated episodes of apparent sinus arrest. However, if a lead becomes disconnected, it may do so at any point in the cardiac cycle, and it is unlikely the onset of 'asystole' will arise after the ventricular T wave as it would if sinus arrest were real. If the onset of sinus arrest does occur during the inscription of an atrial or ventricular complex, artefact can be assumed.

Occasionally, artefact can produce an apparent tachycardia but close inspection will reveal that normal QRS complexes are 'walking through' the tachycardia.

INTERMITTENT ECG RECORDING

Event recorders

Patients with infrequent symptoms are unlikely to experience an episode during a 24-h recording. A very useful and relatively inexpensive device (cardio-memo recorder) enables a patient to record the ECG for 30 s during symptoms. The patient can carry the device around until an attack occurs. He or she then applies the device to the chest wall and initiates the recording, which is stored in a memory and can be replayed directly or transmitted via the telephone into an ECG machine. A similar device which is worn like a wrist-watch is also available. Clearly, these devices are not suitable for the investigation of episodes that disable the patient to the extent that they cannot activate the recorder. It is very important to explain to the patient precisely when and how to use the recorder.

More recently, a small device has become available which can be worn for up to 7 days. Arrhythmias that the device detects and rhythms when the patient activates an event marker can be stored in memory. Importantly, the heart rhythm immediately prior to a symptomatic or detected event is also saved.

Implantable loop recorder

An implantable ECG loop recorder is now available. It is a very small device which can easily be implanted subcutaneously, a few inches below the left clavicle. It facilitates ECG monitoring for up to 18 months and is therefore ideal for patients with infrequent symptoms. After the patient experiences typical symptoms, an external device can be held over the implanted recorder which activates storing of the ECG before, during and after the event. Depending on how the implanted device is programmed, the patient may have up to 30 min after the event to initiate the recording. Thus, the ECG of an arrhythmia which has caused temporary incapacity can be recorded. Memory is sufficient to save ECGs relating to several events. The data can then be downloaded into a computer for analysis.

The latest devices also automatically record the ECG below or above a pre-determined heart rate. Though this facility will ensure that major arrhythmias are stored even if the patient fails to use the external activating device, there is the disadvantage that arrhythmias may be recorded which do not coincide with symptoms and may be of doubtful significance.

Main points

- Ambulatory electrocardiography is very useful for the investigation of syncope, near-syncope, palpitation and other symptoms thought to be due to an arrhythmia when routine electrocardiography has not provided diagnostic information.

- Artefact can produce apparent arrhythmias but can usually be recognized by careful inspection of the recording.

- Studies in apparently normal subjects have demonstrated that certain rhythm disturbances detected by ambulatory electrocardiography are not of pathological significance.

- For patients with infrequent, nondisabling palpitation, provision of an event recorder is the best method of investigation.

- An implantable loop recorder can facilitate ECG recording in patients with infrequent episodes.

- Useful information will be provided from an ambulatory recording if an arrhythmia is demonstrated or if a patient experiences his or her usual symptoms without a disturbance in rhythm. Clearly if there is no arrhythmia and no symptoms, an episodic arrhythmia has not been excluded.

CHAPTER 23

Temporary cardiac pacing

The transvenous route is usually used for temporary pacing but, in emergencies, transcutaneous and oesophageal approaches are possible short-term alternatives.

Temporary transvenous pacing is a simple procedure. However, complications are common because it is often carried out by inexperienced unsupervised operators. The need for temporary pacing should be carefully considered before proceeding.

INDICATIONS

MYOCARDIAL INFARCTION

1. Second- and third-degree AV block due to acute anterior myocardial infarction.
2. Second- and third-degree AV block caused by acute inferior infarction only when complicated by hypotension, ventricular tachyarrhythmia or a ventricular rate less than 40 beats/min.
3. Symptomatic sinus arrest or junctional bradycardia due to acute myocardial infarction.

CHRONIC CONDUCTION TISSUE DISEASE

Temporary pacing may be necessary as a first measure in patients with recent syncope caused by chronic disease of the sinus node or AV junction who are to be referred for long-term pacing.

TACHYCARDIAS

Pacing is useful in terminating AV re-entrant tachycardia, atrial flutter and ventricular tachycardia. In the bradycardia–tachycardia syndrome, temporary pacing should be used to cover cardioversion if required for the termination of supraventricular arrhythmias.

METHODS

TEMPORARY TRANSVENOUS PACING

Temporary ventricular pacing is carried out by introducing a transvenous pacing electrode under local anaesthesia into a systemic vein and advancing it, with the aid of X-ray screening, to the right ventricle. The electrode is connected to an external battery powered pulse generator. During insertion, the heart rhythm must be monitored and equipment for resuscitation should be available.

Subclavian vein puncture

Puncture of the subclavian vein provides the most suitable route of access to the venous system. The vein runs behind the medial third of the clavicle and can be punctured using either supraventricular or infraclavicular approaches. Only the latter will be described.

The patient should lie flat or, if possible, in a slight head-down position. Alternatively, the legs should be raised to aid venous return and hence distension of the subclavian vein. A needle is introduced, through a ½-cm skin incision just below the inferior border of the clavicle and slightly medial to the mid-clavicular point, and is directed towards the sternoclavicular joint so it passes immediately behind the posterior surface of the clavicle. When first advancing the needle it is advisable to locate the clavicle with the needle tip to avoid going in too deeply, with consequent risk of pneumothorax or subclavian artery puncture.

As the needle punctures the vein, venous blood will be easily aspirated. If there is only a trickle of blood, the needle tip is unlikely to be in the subclavian vein.

Cannulation of the vein is best achieved by introducing a guide wire through the needle into the vein. A guide wire with a flexible J-shaped tip is much easier to advance around the junction between the subclavian vein and superior vena cava. The needle is then withdrawn and a sheath within which there is a vessel dilator is passed over the wire into the vein. The guide wire and dilator are then removed, and the pacing lead is passed through the sheath.

The main advantages of subclavian vein puncture are that it is quick and infection and electrode displacement are unusual. Possible complications, which are rare in experienced hands, are pneumothorax, haemothorax, subclavian artery puncture and air embolism.

Antecubital vein cut-down

It is important to select a medially situated vein. It is unusual to be able to negotiate an electrode into the superior vena cava from a lateral vein.

The disadvantages of this approach are poor electrode stability, and infection and phlebitis are common. It may be safer to use this approach in patients who have received thrombolytic therapy.

Femoral vein puncture

This method is very easy and quick, provided that pulsation of the laterally adjacent femoral artery is easily palpable. However, it should be reserved for short-term emergency purposes because electrode stability is poor and there is a risk of venous thrombosis. The femoral vein is medial to the femoral artery. Pressure on the abdomen causes distension of the femoral vein and makes venepuncture easier.

Positioning of the electrode

If there is resistance to the introduction of the electrode into the vein, the lumen has not been entered. Once in the venous system, it should be possible to advance the electrode without resistance. If an obstruction is encountered, the electrode should be withdrawn slightly, rotated and then advanced again. Nothing will be achieved by forcing the electrode.

Once the electrode has reached the right atrium, a loop should be formed by impinging the electrode tip on the atrial wall (Figure 23.1A) and then advancing the electrode a little further (Figure 23.lB). By twisting the electrode, the loop can be rotated so the electrode tip lies near the tricuspid valve (Figure 23.lC). Slight withdrawal of the electrode will allow the tip to 'flick' through the valve into the right ventricle.

Ventricular ectopic beats are usually provoked as the valve is crossed. If these do not occur, the coronary sinus rather than the right ventricle may have been entered. An electrode lying in the coronary sinus assumes a characteristic shape (Figure 23.lF). (A lateral view will show the electrode is pointing posteriorly, whereas an electrode in the right ventricular apex points anteriorly.) It can be confirmed that the right ventricle has been entered by advancing the electrode into the pulmonary artery (Figure 23.lD).

Once in the right ventricle, the electrode tip is positioned in or near the apex of the ventricle by a process of advancement, withdrawal and rotation (Figure 23.lE).

Pacing

When a stable electrode position in or near the right ventricular apex has been achieved, the distal and proximal poles of the electrode should be connected to the pacemaker cathode (–) and anode (+), respectively. If the poles are reversed, the stimulation threshold will be substantially higher.

The pacing threshold, which is the minimum voltage necessary for pacing stimuli to capture the ventricles consistently, should then be measured (Figure 23.2). It

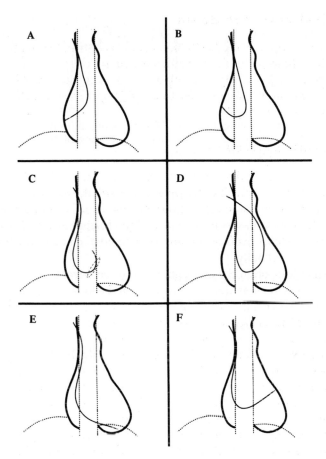

Figure 23.1 Insertion of a transvenous pacing lead. A loop is formed in the right atrium (A and B). The loop is positioned near the tricuspid valve, indicated by the oval of dashes (C). Entry into the right ventricle can be confirmed by passing the wire into the pulmonary artery (D). The pacing lead is then positioned in the apex of the right ventricle (E). (F) The characteristic appearance of a pacing lead in the coronary sinus

should be less than 1.0 V, assuming the pulse generator delivers impulses whose duration is 1 or 2 ms. Some temporary pacemakers allow adjustment of the pulse width: shorter pulse durations lead to a higher threshold and are not indicated for temporary pacing. If the threshold is high, the electrode should be repositioned.

Sometimes, in an emergency, a pacing threshold or electrode position which is less than optimal has to be accepted. Occasionally a patient may become dependent on the pacemaker, making adjustment of the electrode position risky. In these circumstances it may be necessary to insert a second pacing electrode (e.g. via the femoral vein) to cover the period of repositioning.

The stability of the pacing lead should be tested by ensuring there is consistent pacing during coughing and deep inspiration. During the latter manoeuvre, if there is the correct amount of slack in the lead, there will be a slight curve in its right atrial portion (Figure 23.1E).

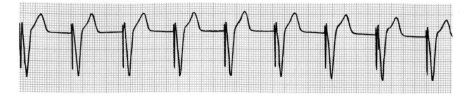

Figure 23.2 Ventricular pacing (lead II). Each pacing stimulus is followed by a ventricular complex. An electrode positioned in the apex of the right ventricle will produce left axis deviation of the paced beats

To avoid lead displacement, it is essential to suture the electrode securely to the skin at its point of entry. The pacing threshold often rises to 2–3 V during the first few days after electrode insertion. The threshold should be checked daily and the output set at twice the measured threshold. Battery and electrical connections should also be checked daily.

It is surprising how often the connections between pacemaker and pacing lead, on which a patient's life may depend, are found to be loose or insecure!

Pacing complications

Causes of failure to pace (Figure 23.3) include electrode displacement, myocardial perforation, exit block and a break in either the electrical connections or in the pacing electrode.

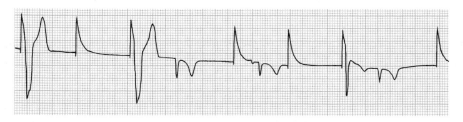

Figure 23.3 Intermittent failure to pace (lead II). Only the first and third pacing stimuli capture the ventricles

ELECTRODE DISPLACEMENT
Electrode displacement may cause intermittent or complete failure to pace. The electrode may fall back into the right atrial cavity and lead to atrial rather than ventricular pacing (Figure 23.4).

MYOCARDIAL PERFORATION
Occasionally the electrode tip may perforate the thin right ventricular myocardium. Failure to pace, diaphragmatic stimulation, pericardial friction rub and pericardial pain may result. Cardiac tamponade is rare.

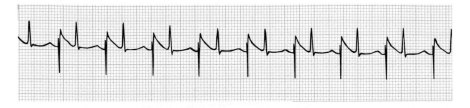

Figure 23.4 Atrial pacing. At the time of this recording, AV conduction was satisfactory so each pacing stimulus was followed by a narrow QRS complex after a PR interval of 0.22 s

Exit block

Sometimes pacing failure occurs without electrode tip displacement or other cause. In these cases failure is attributed to 'exit block', which is caused by excessive tissue reaction at the junction between electrode tip and endocardium.

Electrical fracture

A break in the electrical connection or in the electrode itself can be the cause of intermittent or complete pacing failure. In contrast to exit block, no pacing stimuli will appear on the ECG.

Inappropriate Inhibition

External inhibition of a demand pacemaker from electromagnetic waves being emitted from electrical equipment can occasionally inhibit a pacemaker and will result in absent pacing stimuli. This problem can be quickly solved by changing the pacemaker to fixed-rate mode.

Failure to sense

Pacemakers are most often used in the 'demand' mode, whereby the pacemaker senses spontaneous cardiac activity and only discharges a stimulus if a spontaneous beat has not occurred within a pre-set period. In some patients, those with myocardial infarction, the signal generated by spontaneous activity may be too small for the pacemaker to sense. As a result, the pacemaker will function in a 'fixed rate' mode and pacing stimuli will be discharged at inappropriate times, and may fall on the T wave of a spontaneous beat (Figure 23.5). This is undesirable in acute myocardial infarction because of the risk of precipitating ventricular fibrillation (Figure 23.6).

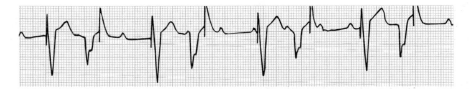

Figure 23.5 Failure to sense in a demand ventricular pacemaker. The first, third, fifth and seventh pacing stimuli capture the ventricles. The second, fourth, sixth and eighth stimuli fall on the T waves of spontaneous ventricular beats

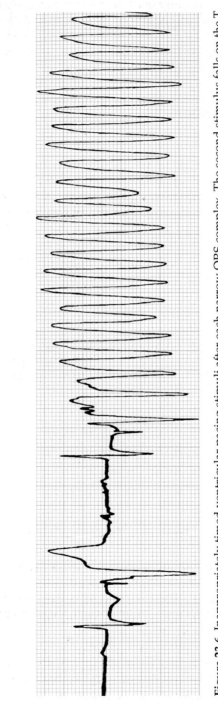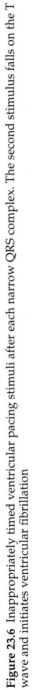

Figure 23.6 Inappropriately timed ventricular pacing stimuli after each narrow QRS complex. The second stimulus falls on the T wave and initiates ventricular fibrillation

INFECTION

Infection can occur at the site of entry of a transvenous pacing electrode. Sometimes bacteraemia results: a serious complication if there is valve disease and thus the possibility of endocarditis. Infection will not clear without removal of the pacing electrode. If necessary, a new pacing electrode will have to be inserted at a different site.

AV SEQUENTIAL PACING

Ventricular pacing results in dissociation between atrial and ventricular activity and a consequent reduction in cardiac output of up to one-third.

The atria and ventricles may be paced sequentially, enabling the normal sequence of cardiac chamber activation (Figure 23.7). In patients with a low cardiac output, AV sequential pacing can produce an important improvement in cardiac function. Usually, AV sequential pacing is achieved by passing two leads to the heart: one to the atria and one to the ventricles. The best method of ensuring that an atrial lead is not displaced is to use one with a pre-formed J-shaped terminal portion. A lead of this type can easily be positioned in the right atrial appendage (*see* chapter 16).

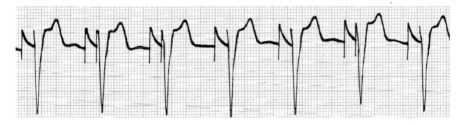

Figure 23.7 AV sequential pacing. Pacing stimuli precede both atrial and ventricular complexes

TEMPORARY TRANSCUTANEOUS AND OESOPHAGEAL PACING

Transcutaneous cardiac pacing was first attempted many years ago but was usually unsuccessful and caused severe discomfort due to skeletal muscle stimulation. Recently, considerable success with less discomfort has been achieved by using large surface area skin electrodes and stimuli of much longer duration than are used for endocardial stimulation (20–40 ms).

The latest generation of transcutaneous pacemakers function in the demand mode and have a maximum output in the region of 150 mA. One electrode is applied to the front of the chest and the other to the back over the right scapula. Pacing is likely to stimulate the atria at the same time as the ventricles. It is not always possible to ascertain from the ECG that the heart is being stimulated: monitoring of an arterial pulse may be necessary.

With oesophageal pacing, a long impulse duration is necessary (10 ms). Atrial stimulation is more successful than ventricular stimulation.

As with transvenous pacing, transcutaneous and oesophageal pacing are unlikely to be successful after a prolonged period of cardiac arrest.

Main points

- Indications for temporary transvenous pacing include: second- and third-degree AV block due to acute anterior infarction; 'complicated' second- and third-degree AV block due to acute inferior infarction; and recent syncope or near-syncope due to chronic disease of the sinus node or AV junction while awaiting implantation of a long-term pacemaker.

- Subclavian vein puncture is usually the best method of venous access for temporary pacing.

- The pacemaker stimulation threshold, battery function and electrical connections should be checked daily.

- AV sequential pacing improves cardiac output as compared with ventricular pacing.

Long-term cardiac pacing for bradycardias

This subject is discussed in detail to provide a concise account of the practical aspects of pacemaker implantation and the care of patients with pacemakers; often the remit of a cardiac department's more junior members.

An artificial cardiac pacemaker generates electrical stimuli which can initiate myocardial contraction. The stimuli are usually delivered to the heart by transvenous leads or much less commonly via epicardial, oesophageal or transthoracic electrodes.

The first pacemaker was implanted in 1958. Over the following years, rapid progress in technology and an increasing awareness of the benefits of pacing have led to pacemakers being widely used. Patients of all ages, from the newborn to over 100 years old, have been paced: the average age at first implantation is 72 years.

INDICATIONS FOR LONG-TERM CARDIAC PACING

The main reasons for implanting a pacemaker are to relieve symptoms or to improve prognosis. In some patients with asymptomatic impairment of the specialized cardiac conducting system, other factors may also be pertinent such as the need for medication which may cause unwanted bradycardia, or concern in a motor vehicle driver that an accident might result should syncope occur.

COMPLETE ATRIOVENTRICULAR BLOCK

Syncope

The most common reason for pacemaker implantation is to prevent syncope or near-syncope due to complete AV block. A single episode is a sufficient indication and since the next blackout may cause injury or be fatal, delay should be minimal. Even in patients with a short life expectancy, pacing should be considered if by preventing syncope, independence may be preserved and serious injury avoided.

Dyspnoea

Complete heart block can reduce cardiac output and thereby cause exertional dyspnoea and sometimes cardiac failure. Pacing usually improves these problems.

Cerebration

Mental impairment is sometimes attributed to heart block but often does not improve with pacing; if there is doubt, it is best to undertake a trial of temporary pacing.

Prognosis

Without pacing, the prognosis in patients with complete heart block is poor. With an artificial pacemaker, life expectancy closely approaches that of the general population though those with overt coronary heart disease or with heart failure have a less good outlook. Pacemaker implantation should be considered in asymptomatic patients with complete AV block, particularly when the ventricular rate is 40 beats/min or less, on purely prognostic grounds.

QRS BREADTH

Narrow ventricular complexes during complete AV block suggests that interruption in conduction is at AV nodal level and that, in contrast to infranodal block, a subsidiary pacemaker within the His bundle will discharge reliably at a relatively rapid ventricular rate. However, in practice, patients with narrow ventricular complexes during complete heart block may experience syncope and impaired exercise tolerance. In the United Kingdom, one-third of patients who receive pacemakers for complete AV block have narrow QRS complexes.

Congenital heart block

Congenital heart block, i.e. complete AV block that is discovered as a neonate or child and is not caused by acquired disease, is widely regarded as benign. However, some patients do develop symptoms or die suddenly. If heart block has caused symptoms then pacing is indicated. In young asymptomatic patients the risks of not implanting a pacemaker have to be weighed against the possibility of complications associated with several decades of pacing. There are several documented risk factors: day-time ventricular rate less than 50 beats/min, broad QRS complexes, pauses more than 3.0 s, frequent ventricular ectopic beats and poor chronotropic response to exercise. Unpaced patients should undergo ambulatory and exercise electrocardiography at regular intervals.

SECOND-DEGREE AV BLOCK

Mobitz II AV block often progresses to complete AV block. The approach to Mobitz II AV block is similar to that for complete AV block.

A study has refuted the previously held view that Mobitz I AV block is benign in that the incidence of symptoms, prognosis and influence of pacing were the same as for patients with Mobitz II block. This poor outlook does not, however, apply to young people with transient and often nocturnal Wenkebach block, which is due to high vagal tone and is benign.

FIRST-DEGREE AV BLOCK

First-degree AV block is not itself an indication for cardiac pacing. If a patient presents with first-degree block and syncope or near-syncope, it is quite possible that the symptoms are due to transient second- or third-degree AV block but a pacemaker should not be implanted without proof of this, e.g. by ambulatory electrocardiography.

BUNDLE BRANCH AND FASCICULAR BLOCKS

Bundle branch block

The risk of high-degree AV block developing in an asymptomatic patient with either left or right bundle branch block is very small, and pacing is not indicated. In patients who present with syncope or near-syncope the approach should be the same as for first-degree AV block.

Bifascicular block

In bifascicular block the remaining functioning fascicle may fail to conduct, intermittently or persistently, and cause high-degree AV block. In patients with a good history of Stokes–Adams attacks, pacemaker implantation is indicated to prevent syncope without further investigation. With atypical symptoms, high-degree AV block must be documented first. Some patients with bifascicular block have been shown to be prone to ventricular tachycardia.

In asymptomatic bifascicular block, the chances of progression to complete AV block is in the order of 2% per year and the major determinants of prognosis are the presence of coronary artery or myocardial disease; prophylactic pacing is generally not indicated. Additional first-degree AV block or His bundle electrographic evidence of prolonged infranodal conduction suggest that conduction in the functioning fascicle is also impaired. However, there is no evidence of a higher risk.

AV and bundle branch block after myocardial infarction

AV block due to inferior myocardial infarction usually resolves within a few days and almost always by 3 weeks. When anterior infarction is complicated by high-degree AV block, there is usually extensive myocardial damage and hence the prognosis is poor: though block may persist it is prudent to ensure that the patient is going to survive before implanting a pacemaker. Thus pacemaker implantation should not be considered unless second- or third-degree AV block is present 3 weeks after myocardial infarction.

When a patient is admitted to hospital with heart block, there is often an unnecessary delay before referral for long-term pacing while myocardial infarction is excluded. Unless the patient has experienced typical cardiac pain or there are typical ECG changes of recent infarction, AV block has probably not been caused by acute infarction.

Bifascicular block persisting after acute anterior infarction complicated by AV block raises the possibility that complete AV block might recur. Intermittent heart block has been demonstrated to occur in some patients with post-infarction bifascicular block and may necessitate pacing. However, there is little evidence that prophylactic pacing reduces mortality.

SICK SINUS SYNDROME

Syncope

Sick sinus syndrome accounts for more than one-third of pacemaker implantations. Pacing is indicated when syncope or near-syncope are caused. It should be remembered that sinus bradycardia and pauses in sinus node activity for up to 3.0 s, particularly if nocturnal, can be physiological.

Bradycardia–tachycardia syndrome

In patients with the bradycardia–tachycardia syndrome, pacing may be required to avoid severe bradycardia caused by anti-arrhythmic drugs. Sometimes atrial tachy-arrhythmias which start during bradycardia will be prevented by atrial pacing. The risk of systemic embolism will thereby be reduced.

Prognosis

Pacing for sick sinus syndrome is not usually indicated in asymptomatic patients. However, pauses in cardiac activity for several seconds might be considered an indication for pacing in those who operate machinery, including a motor car, to avoid an accident should syncope occur.

HYPERSENSITIVE CAROTID SINUS AND MALIGNANT VASOVAGAL SYNDROMES

Pacing will improve symptoms in these syndromes provided there is a significant cardioinhibitory component (*see* chapter 17).

HYPERTROPHIC OBSTRUCTIVE CARDIOMYOPATHY

Dual-chambered pacing with a short AV delay has been shown to reduce symptoms and left ventricular outflow tract gradient in some patients with hypertrophic obstructive cardiomyopathy.

RESYNCHRONIZATION THERAPY

Recently, biventricular pacing has been shown to improve symptoms in patients with poor left ventricular function who have marked prolongation of QRS duration, usually due to left bundle branch block. The left ventricle is activated simultaneously by stimuli conducted via right and left ventricular leads, usually resulting in significant shortening of QRS duration. Left ventricular pacing is achieved by passing an additional lead into a lateral branch of the coronary sinus.

PACING MODES

The first generation of pacemakers functioned in a fixed-rate mode: the pacemaker stimulated the ventricles regularly, usually at 70 beats/min, irrespective of any spontaneous cardiac activity (Figure 24.1). Competition with a spontaneous rhythm could cause irregular palpitation (Figure 24.2), and stimulation during ventricular repolarization could possibly initiate ventricular fibrillation (*see* Figure 23.6).

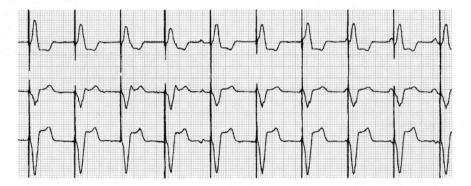

Figure 24.1 Fixed-rate ventricular pacing (leads I, II, III). A large pacing stimulus precedes each ventricular complex

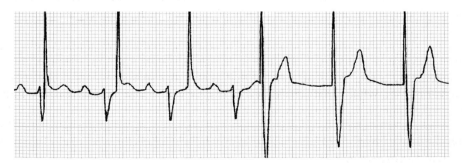

Figure 24.2 Fixed-rate ventricular pacing in a patient with first-degree AV block. The first three stimuli fall during the refractory period and are ineffective. The fourth causes a premature contraction

Subsequent developments enabled sensing of spontaneous activity via the stimulating lead to facilitate demand pacing: a sensed event resets the timing of delivery of the next pacemaker stimulus to avoid competition with spontaneous activity (Figure 24.3).

With the advent of reliable atrial transvenous pacing leads it became straightforward to pace and sense in the atrium as well as the ventricle, thus allowing both atrial and ventricular 'single-chamber' pacing and also 'dual-chamber' pacing whereby stimulation and/or sensing can take place at both atrial and ventricular levels. These developments have permitted a more physiological approach to cardiac stimulation.

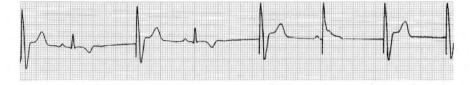

Figure 24.3 Demand ventricular pacemaker. The pacemaker is inhibited by the sinus beats (second and fourth complexes). The sixth complex is a fusion beat. A 'P' wave can be seen to precede the pacing stimulus. By chance, a sinus impulse has arisen at the instant when the pacemaker was set to discharge and the ventricles have been activated by both stimulus impulse and pacemaker. Fusion beats should not be confused with failure to pace

PACING SYSTEM CODE

A five-letter code is widely used to describe the various pacing modes.

The first character identifies the chamber or chambers that are paced: 'A' for atrium, 'V' for ventricle and 'D' (for dual), if both atrium and ventricle can be stimulated.

The second character indicates the chamber or chambers whose activity is sensed: in addition to the use of 'A', 'V' and 'D', 'O' indicates that the pacemaker is insensitive.

The third character denotes the response to the sensed information. 'I' indicates that pacemaker output is inhibited by a sensed event, 'T' that stimulation is triggered by a sensed event and 'D' that ventricular sensed events inhibit pacemaker output, while atrial-sensed events trigger ventricular stimulation. 'O' indicates that there is no response to sensed events.

A fourth character, 'R', is used if there is a rate-responsive facility whereby the pacing rate is modulated by a sensor that detects a physiological variable such as activity or respiration.

The fifth character only relates to anti-tachycardia pacemakers: 'O', none; 'P', anti-tachycardia pacing (low-energy stimulation); 'S', shock (i.e. cardioversion or defibrillation); and 'D', both anti-tachycardia pacing and shock.

SINGLE-CHAMBER PACING

Ventricular demand pacing (VVI)

In the absence of spontaneous ventricular activity, a ventricular demand pace-maker, like a fixed-rate unit, delivers stimuli to the ventricles at a regular rate. However, if spontaneous activity is sensed via the ventricular lead, the timing of delivery of the next pacemaker output is reset to avoid competition.

In ventricular inhibited pacemakers (VVI), a sensed event terminates the current stimulation cycle, thus inhibiting pacemaker output, and starts a new cycle (Figure 24.3). In contrast, a sensed event during the less commonly used mode of ventricular triggered (VVT) pacing immediately triggers delivery of a pacing stimulus which will consequently fall during the myocardial refractory period and will thus be ineffective. The subsequent cycle will then start from delivery of the triggered impulsive (Figure 24.4).

The pacemaker is rendered insensitive immediately after a paced or sensed event for an interval, which approximates the duration of myocardial activation and recovery to prevent sensing the ventricular electrogram which is produced by the event. This interval (250–300 ms) is referred to as the refractory period.

Ventricular demand pacing is a commonly employed mode but its use is diminishing now that its disadvantages – the inability to facilitate the normal sequence of cardiac chamber activation and to provide a chronotropic response to exercise – are widely appreciated (see below).

Indications for ventricular demand pacing include bradycardia associated with persistent atrial fibrillation, second- and third-degree AV block in patients who are limited by impaired cerebral or locomotor function and patients with infrequent bradycardia in whom the pacemaker is mainly on 'stand-by'.

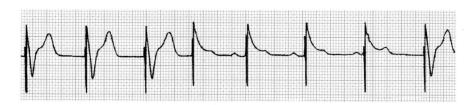

Figure 24.4 Ventricular triggered pacemaker. After the first three paced beats there is sinus rhythm. A pacing stimulus is discharged immediately after the onset of the QRS complex in these beats

Atrial demand pacing (AAI)

The timing cycles of atrial inhibited (AAI) and the less commonly used atrial triggered (AAT) modes are the same as for ventricular demand pacing, as described above (Figure 24.5). With atrial pacing, the refractory period is usually longer to avoid inappropriate inhibition of the pacemaker by sensing the 'far-field' ventricular electrogram via the atrial lead.

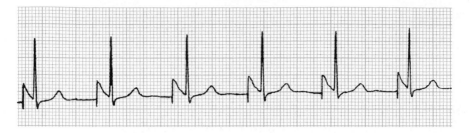

Figure 24.5 Atrial pacing. A pacing stimulus precedes each P wave.

Atrial pacing is indicated for treatment of the sick sinus syndrome unless AV conduction is impaired. By stimulating the atria rather than the ventricles, the normal sequence of cardiac chamber activation is maintained, loss of which can reduce cardiac output by up to one-third.

Sick sinus syndrome can sometimes be associated with impaired AV conduction. However, if there is no evidence of it at the time of pacemaker implantation, the subsequent development of impaired AV conduction is uncommon. Dual-chamber pacing is indicated if there is also bifascicular or bundle branch block or if, during pacemaker implantation, atrial pacing at a rate of 120 beats/min causes second-degree AV block.

DUAL-CHAMBER PACING

AV sequential pacing (DVI and DDI)

In AV sequential (DVI) pacing the atria are stimulated first and then, after a delay which approximates the normal PR interval, the ventricles are stimulated (Figure 24.6). The pacemaker is inhibited by spontaneous ventricular activity but no sensing occurs in the atrium. As with other dual-chamber modes, both atrial and ventricular electrodes are required.

Fusion beats (Figure 24.7) are commonly seen during DVI pacing and are sometimes misinterpreted as pacemaker malfunction: whereas the pacemaker is inhibited by an event sensed in the ventricles, the first chamber to be stimulated is the atrium. Pacemaker output may therefore occur at the same time as spontaneous atrial activation because its resultant ventricular depolarisation has not yet occurred.

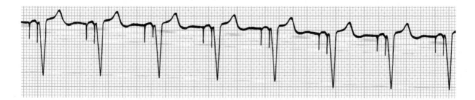

Figure 24.6 AV sequential (DVI) pacing. Pacing stimuli precede both atrial and ventricular complexes

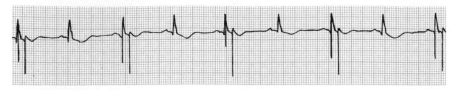

Figure 24.7 DVI pacing: fusion beats

More recently, the mode of DDI pacing has been introduced. Sensing occurs at atrial as well as ventricular levels, thus avoiding competitive atrial pacing. Unlike DDD pacing, sensed atrial events do not trigger ventricular stimulation and thus this mode cannot facilitate endless loop tachycardia (see below).

The main indications for DVI and DDI pacing are sick sinus syndrome associated with impaired AV conduction, and carotid sinus and malignant vasovagal syndromes.

Atrial synchronized ventricular pacing (VDD)

In this mode, ventricular stimulation is triggered by a sensed atrial event after an interval similar to the normal PR interval (Figure 24.8). It thereby maintains the normal sequence of cardiac chamber activation and permits a chronotropic response to exercise provided sinus node function is normal.

If an atrial event is not sensed, ventricular stimulation continues at a fixed cycle length – otherwise atrial standstill might lead to ventricular asystole. To avoid atrial tachycardia or fibrillation triggering inappropriately fast ventricular pacing rates, there is an atrial refractory interval: the atrial channel is rendered insensitive during the AV delay and for a period after ventricular stimulation. Sensed atrial activity at a cycle length shorter than this period will not trigger ventricular stimulation.

The upper rate at which atrial activity will trigger ventricular output is determined by the 'total atrial refractory period', which consists of the AV delay plus the post-ventricular stimulus refractory period. For example, if the AV delay is 125 ms and the atrial refractory period is 250 ms, the upper rate limit will be 60 000/375 = 160 beats/min.

In earlier years, sensing only took place in the atrium and pacing only occurred in the ventricle (VAT). Thus ventricular ectopic beats or rhythms faster than the sinus node rate would not inhibit ventricular output. Subsequently, VDD pacing was introduced whereby sensing takes place in the ventricles as well so that spontaneous ventricular activity will inhibit the pacemaker (Figure 24.9).

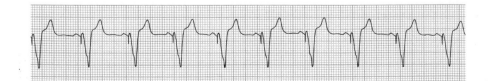

Figure 24.8 Atrial synchronized pacing. Each P wave triggers a paced ventricular beat

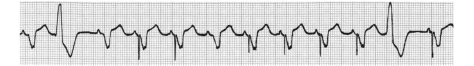

Figure 24.9 VDD pacing, showing chronotropic response to exercise and inhibition by ventricular ectopic beats

Atrial synchronized ventricular pacing is indicated in second- and third-degree AV block when sinus node function is normal. It is contraindicated in sick sinus syndrome or when there are atrial tachyarrhythmias.

Endless loop tachycardia

If a ventricular stimulus is conducted retrogradely to the atria via either the AV junction or, if present, an accessory AV pathway, and the timing of the resultant atrial activation is outside the pacemaker's atrial refractory period, it will trigger ventricular stimulation and hence initiate an 'endless loop tachycardia' (Figure 24.10), also referred to as 'pacemaker-mediated tachycardia'.

Ventriculo-atrial conduction is present in approximately two-thirds of patients with sick sinus syndrome and one-fifth of those with complete AV block. Endless loop tachycardia can usually be prevented by prolongation of the atrial refractory period but at the expense of reduction of the upper rate limit for ventricular stimulation. Endless loop tachycardia can be avoided in 90% of patients by setting the AV delay to 125 ms and the post-ventricular atrial refractory period to 300 ms.

Most pacemakers can detect endless loop tachycardia and interrupt it, for example, by prolonging the atrial refractory period for one cycle.

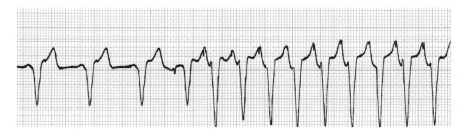

Figure 24.10 Pacemaker-mediated tachycardia after four cycles of dual-chambered pacing

AV universal pacing (DDD)

In this mode (DDD), which all modern dual-chamber pacemakers can facilitate, both sensing and pacing can take place at atrial and ventricular levels. Universal pacing allows the pacemaker to function in atrial demand (AAI), AV sequential (DVI, DDI) or atrial synchronized (VDD) modes depending on the spontaneous heart rhythm (Figure 24.11).

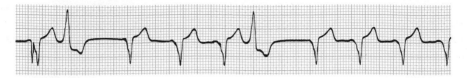

Figure 24.11 Universal (DDD) pacing. Spontaneous P waves trigger ventricular stimulation. After the first and fifth paced beats there are ventricular ectopic beats which inhibit the pacemaker. There is sinus node depression following the ectopics to which the pacemaker responds by pacing the atria as well as the ventricles

If there is sinus bradycardia, it functions as an atrial demand pacemaker. If there is impaired AV conduction, ventricular pacing is triggered by either spontaneous atrial activity or by delivery of an atrial stimulus. When sinus node function is normal, it functions in the atrial synchronized mode, thus providing a chronotropic response to exercise. The pacemaker is inhibited by both atrial and ventricular ectopic beats. Endless loop tachycardia may occur if there is retrograde AV conduction.

DDD pacing is indicated in second- and third-degree AV block. Atrial tachyarrhythmias are a contraindication because the rapid atrial rate would trigger an inappropriately fast ventricular pacing.

'PHYSIOLOGICAL PACING'

Physiological pacing systems facilitate a chronotropic response to exercise by maintaining atrioventricular synchronization as the sinus node rate varies and/or by a rate adaptive mechanism.

Atrial synchronized ventricular pacing

This mode, which both maintains AV synchronization and facilitates a chronotropic response, has been shown to increase cardiac output at rest and during exercise as compared with ventricular pacing. Exercise capacity has been measured on a double-blind basis during ventricular pacing at 70 beats/min and during atrial synchronized ventricular pacing. The latter mode has been demonstrated to increase maximal exercise capacity by approximately 30%. However, individual patients varied in the degree by which they benefited: in a few there was little improvement, whereas in many there was a dramatic increase. Neither age nor cause of heart block predicted the amount of benefit. It used to be thought that 'physiological' pacing was of greatest value to patients with poor ventricular function. This is not the case; indeed, patients with high venous pressures may not benefit.

Atrial synchronized pacing improves parameters in addition to maximal exercise tolerance. Shortness of breath, dizziness and palpitation are less frequent whereas fixed rate pacing tends to impair the normal blood pressure response to exercise, and leads to a higher respiratory rate and perceived exertion during submaximal exercise. The advantages of atrial synchronized pacing have been shown to be maintained in the long term.

There are limitations to atrial synchronized ventricular pacing. First, normal or at least near-normal sinus node activity is required. Secondly, the ventricular stimulation rate may increase in response to an atrial tachyarrhythmia. Thirdly, an atrial as well as a ventricular pacing lead is required.

Rate response systems

Several pacing systems are available that can facilitate a chronotropic response independent of atrial activity: a change in stimulation rate is achieved in response to a parameter that alters with exercise. In contrast to atrial synchronized pacing, normal sinus node activity is not required.

In terms of exercise capacity, the ability to increase heart rate is far more important than maintaining atrioventricular synchronization. This has been demonstrated by measuring exercise tolerance during three pacing modes: fixed rate, atrial synchronized, and ventricular pacing at a rate equal to but not synchronized with atrial activity. Both the latter forms of chronotropic pacing increased exercise performance to a similar degree as compared with fixed-rate pacing. Thus rate response ventricular pacemakers can enable an enhanced exercise tolerance without the need for an atrial lead.

Some patients with sick sinus syndrome have chronotropic incompetence: there is little increase in sinus node rate in response to exercise. A rate-responsive system will facilitate an appropriate rate response.

According to the pacemaker code, a ventricular demand and a dual-chambered pacemaker with a rate response facility are termed VVIR and DDDR, respectively.

ACTIVITY SENSOR
Vibration resulting from physical activity is sensed by a piezoelectric crystal attached to the inside of the pacemaker can or an accelerometer bonded to the circuitry within the pacemaker. The stimulation rate increases in parallel with the level of sensed activity. An accelerometer is regarded as more physiological since it will respond to motion primarily in the anteroposterior direction. The systems have been criticized because they are not truly physiological. For example, the same levels of vibration and hence the same heart rate will be generated by ascending and descending a flight of stairs though less work is required for the latter. There will be no response to nonexertional stresses such as emotion or illness. In addition, in the case of a piezoelectrical crystal, the pacemaker rate may increase in response to pressure on the pacemaker can itself. However, in contrast to systems using other sensors, a very prompt and reliable chronotropic response to exercise is achieved.

EVOKED QT RESPONSE
Though it has been known for many years that the QT interval decreases with increasing heart rate, it has only recently been appreciated that sympathetic nervous system activity is a major independent determinant of QT interval duration: QT interval shortens during exercise even during fixed rate pacing. The pacemaker senses, via a conventional ventricular pacing electrode, the interval between pacing stimulus and apex of the elicited T wave: a decrease in the interval leads to an increase in stimulation rate.

Since this system responds to sympathetic nervous system activity, it will increase the heart rate in response to emotion as well as exertion.

RESPIRATION
There is a close relation between minute volume and heart rate. The system's discharge rate is governed by changes in intravascular impedance, a measure of respiratory minute volume, which is monitored by means of a conventional bipolar pacing lead.

BLOOD TEMPERATURE
Skeletal muscle activity generates heat which is transferred to the blood. There is a relation between level of exercise and right ventricular blood temperature. One problem, however, is that there is a latency in the system due to the delay of 1 or 2 min before blood temperature rises after the start of exercise.

OTHER SENSORS
Other parameters such as oxygen saturation and right ventricular pressure are being investigated for use in rate-response pacing. Information on long-term reliability of sensors is not yet available. Rate-response systems that can use a conventional lead have practical advantages over systems that require a lead incorporating a specialized sensor.

MULTISENSOR PACING
Dual-chamber pacemakers are available which, in addition to sensing atrial activity, will respond to parameters related to exercise such as activity or QT interval (DDDR). Thus, normal AV synchrony can be maintained and a chronotropic response to exercise can be provided even if sinus node function is impaired or if an intermittent atrial arrhythmia occurs.

Some newer pacing systems incorporate not one but two types of physiological sensor so that the limitations of each system can be minimized. For example, an activity sensor to provide a prompt response and a QT sensor to ensure the rate response is proportional to the workload.

Automatic mode switching

This relatively new facility allows implantation of DDD pacemaker in patients prone to paroxysmal atrial fibrillation and other atrial tachyarrhythmias. When rapid, abnormal atrial activity is sensed, the pacing mode automatically switches from DDD or DDDR to VVI or VVIR, respectively. Dual-chamber pacing resumes on termination of the atrial arrhythmia (Figure 24.12).

'Pacemaker syndrome'

It is at rest that the disadvantage of loss of AV synchrony caused by ventricular pacing may become apparent. Atrial contraction may occur against closed mitral and tricuspid valves. Atrial pressure will rise and impede venous return so that during the next diastolic period the ventricles will be underfilled with resultant reduction in

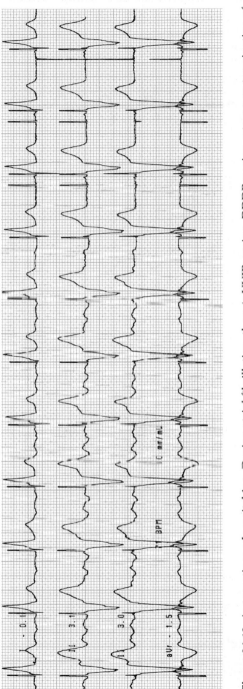
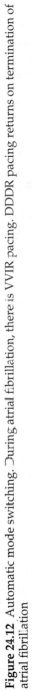

Figure 24.12 Automatic mode switching. During atrial fibrillation, there is VVIR pacing. DDDR pacing returns on termination of atrial fibrillation

stroke volume. Loss of properly timed atrial systole reduces cardiac output by up to one-third and may cause hypotension: near-syncope and syncope can result (Figure 24.13). Other symptoms include weakness, dizziness and dyspnoea. Ventricul-oatrial conduction (Figure 24.14) causes even greater haemodynamic upset: the resultant atrial distension may initiate a reflex vasodepressor effect.

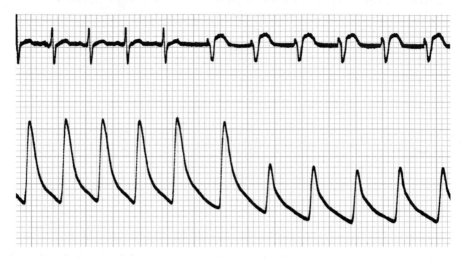

Figure 24.13 Pacemaker syndrome. There was symptomatic hypotension (lower trace) during ventricular pacing which occurs after the first four sinus beats

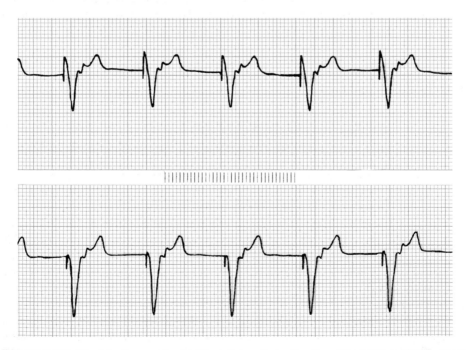

Figure 24.14 Ventricular pacing with retrograde activation (leads II and III). Each ventricular complex is followed by an inverted P wave

Hypotension is likely to be more marked whilst standing. It is most severe during the first few seconds of ventricular pacing, before vasoconstrictor compensatory mechanisms can come into play, so ventricular pacing is particularly unsuitable for patients who are mainly in sinus rhythm but who often develop bradycardia at a rate less than the cycle length of the ventricular pacemaker, i.e. those with sick sinus or carotid sinus syndromes. This has been demonstrated by recording ambulatory blood pressure in patients with ventricular demand pacemakers. The onset of ventricular pacing was followed by hypotension which was greater in those who had complained of syncope and near-syncope. Atrioventricular sequential pacing or, when AV conduction is not impaired, atrial pacing will avoid these problems.

PACEMAKER HARDWARE

PULSE GENERATOR

A pulse generator consists of a power source together with electronic circuits to control the timing and characteristics of the impulses that it generates.

In the past, several power sources have been used, including mercury–zinc cells, rechargeable nickel cadmium cells and nuclear energy. Now, lithium iodide cells are used almost exclusively. Lithium pacemakers have a life span of 4–15 years and a predictable, progressive discharge behaviour. They are contained in a hermetically sealed titanium can, 35–50 g in weight, and generally have a maximum diameter of no more than 50 mm and a thickness of as little as 6 mm.

PACEMAKER LEADS

Stimuli produced by the pulse generator are conducted to the heart via a lead, which consists of an insulated wire with an electrode at its tip which is attached to the heart.

Transvenous leads are used in over 95% of pacemaker implantations. A modern lead consists of a multifilar, helically coiled wire which is insulated by a material that does not cause tissue reaction or thrombosis: silicone rubber or polyurethane. At the lead tip is the cathode which is composed of an inert material such as platinum–iridium, elgiloy, steel or vitreous carbon. For effective stimulation, this must be securely and closely attached to the endocardium. If fibrous tissue, which is nonexcitable, develops between cathode and endocardium, the amount of energy required to stimulate the heart will increase and may exceed the output capability of the pacemaker.

To achieve a low threshold for stimulation and secure endocardial attachment, several 'fixation devices' have been employed. 'Passive' fixation devices include tines, flanges or fins positioned proximal to the lead tip which can become entrapped in the myocardial trabeculae. 'Active' devices include an electrode in the shape of a helix which by rotation of the lead can be wound around a trabeculum, and a retractable metal screw which can be screwed into the endo-myocardium. 'Porous' metal or carbon electrodes are now widely used; the surface of the cathode consists of many microscopic pores which promote rapid tissue ingrowth and hence very secure fixation. Movement between electrode and endocardium and thus generation of fibrous tissue is minimized. Many types of electrode elute dexamethasone to minimize local tissue reaction and hence stimulation threshold.

Attachment of atrial leads was impracticable until the advent of fixation devices. The distal portion of atrial leads are often 'J' shaped to facilitate positioning in the right atrial appendage.

The amount of energy required to stimulate the heart is related to the surface area of the cathode. Nowadays, low surface area electrodes are used – 6–12 mm^2.

Leads that are sewn on to the epicardium or screwed into the myocardium necessitate thoracotomy. With the advent of reliable transvenous leads, they are now rarely used unless pacemaker implantation is undertaken at the time of open heart surgery, or venous thrombosis or tricuspid valve prosthesis preclude a transvenous approach.

Unipolar versus bipolar pacing

In unipolar pacing the anode is remote from the heart; usually the metal can containing the pulse generator. In bipolar pacing, both anode and cathode are within the cardiac chamber to be paced, with the anode positioned along the lead near to its cathodal tip. A commonly held view is that an electrogram sensed by a unipolar lead is larger than that from a bipolar lead. There is in fact usually no difference between bipolar and unipolar electrograms or stimulation thresholds.

Bipolar pacing has the advantage that inappropriate sensing of electromagnetic interference and skeletal muscle electromyograms is much less likely, as is extracardiac stimulation. Reasons for favouring unipolar pacing are that there is greater experience with unipolar leads, in the past bipolar electrodes have been less reliable and larger in calibre, and surface ECG unipolar pacemaker stimuli are larger, making ECG interpretation easier.

Costs

In the United Kingdom, the current approximate costs of a pulse generator plus leads for single-chamber and dual-chambered pacing systems are £800 and £1500, respectively.

PACEMAKER IMPLANTATION

Facilities for fluoroscopy, ECG monitoring and cardiopulmonary resuscitation are required. The procedure is usually carried out under local anaesthesia and takes 15–45 min.

SUBCLAVIAN APPROACH

The subclavian approach is now widely used and is especially useful if more than one lead is to be inserted. The pacemaker lead(s) are introduced via infraclavicular subclavian vein puncture and are connected to the pulse generator, which is implanted in a subcutaneous pocket fashioned over pectoralis major.

An incision is made 2 cm below the junction of the middle and inner thirds of the clavicle and is extended in a lateral and usually inferior direction for approximately 6 cm. A subcutaneous pocket large enough to accommodate the pulse generator is created by blunt dissection.

Puncture of the subclavian vein is easier if the vein is distended: a slight head-down position will help or, alternatively, the legs should be raised. Dehydration should be corrected. A needle is introduced just below the inferior border of the clavicle at the junction of its middle and inner thirds and directed towards the sternoclavicular joint so that it passes behind the posterior surface of the clavicle. As the needle punctures the vein, venous blood will be aspirated easily; only a trickle suggests that the needle is not in the vein. Aspiration of air or bright pulsatile blood indicate puncture of the pleura or subclavian artery, respectively. If the patient has a 'deep' chest, and particularly if the clavicle bows anteriorly, it may be necessary to introduce the needle a little more laterally and to point it slightly posteriorly.

Cannulation of the vein is then achieved by introducing a flexible guide wire, preferably with a J-shaped tip, through the needle. Resistance to its passage indicates that the wire is not in the vein. The wire is passed into the superior vena cava and its position checked by fluoroscopy. The needle is then withdrawn and a sheath within which is a vessel dilator is passed over the wire into the vein. The guidewire and dilator are then removed and the pacing lead inserted into the sheath. If it is planned to introduce a second pacing lead, then the guidewire can be left in place to permit introduction of a second introducer and sheath. 'Peel-away' sheaths are used so that their removal is not prevented by the connector at the proximal end of the lead.

Cephalic vein approach

An alternative to subclavian vein puncture is to cut down on to the cephalic vein in the deltopectoral groove. This approach avoids the risks of subclavian vein puncture, but the vein may not be large enough to accommodate two leads and sometimes is even too small for one lead. It can sometimes be difficult to advance a lead from the cephalic into the subclavian vein.

POSITIONING OF A VENTRICULAR LEAD

To facilitate manipulation of a long-term pacing lead, which is very flexible, a wire stylet is passed down the centre of the lead. Bending the distal part of the stylet or slight withdrawal will often aid positioning. The lead is passed into the right atrium (see Figure 23.1). Sometimes the lead can then be directly advanced through the tricuspid valve to the right ventricular apex. More often, it is necessary to form a loop in the atrium by impinging the lead tip on the atrial wall and then advancing the lead a little further. By rotating the lead its tip can then be positioned near the tricuspid valve. Slight withdrawal of the lead will allow it to 'flick' through the valve into the ventricle. Ventricular ectopic beats are almost always provoked as the valve is crossed. If these do not occur, then the coronary sinus may have been entered.

Entry into the ventricle can be confirmed by advancing the lead into the pulmonary artery. Once in the right ventricle, the lead tip is positioned in or near the ventricular apex by a process of lead rotation, advancement and withdrawal. A stable position should be ensured by checking for continuous pacing and for absence of excessive lead tip movement during deep inspiration and coughing. Once a satisfactory position has been achieved both in terms of stability and measurements (see below), it is essential that the lead is secured by placing a short length of rubber sleeve around it near its point of entry into the vein and fixing it to the underlying muscle with a nonadsorbable suture.

Recently, there has been interest in pacing the right ventricular outflow tract rather than apex. There is evidence of haemodynamic advantage in some patients and no evidence of harm. An active fixation lead is required.

POSITIONING OF AN ATRIAL LEAD

The right atrial appendage is the usual site for atrial pacing. If necessary, atrial pacing may be performed by using a 'screw-in' lead to pace from the septal or free right atrial walls.

For pacing the right atrial appendage, a lead with a J-shaped terminal portion is usually used. First, using a straight stylet, the lead tip is straightened and advanced to the mid-right atrium. The lead is then rotated so that its tip is near the tricuspid valve. Partial withdrawal of the stylet causes the lead to assume its J shape and slight withdrawal of the lead itself allows the lead tip to enter the appendage. A straight lead may be positioned in the appendage by use of a stylet whose terminal 2–3 inches have been shaped into a tight 'J'.

Correct positioning will be demonstrated by the lead tip moving from side to side with atrial systole. Lateral screening will demonstrate that the lead is pointing anteriorly. Lead stability should be confirmed by twisting the lead 45 degrees in either direction; the lead tip should not turn. It is important that there is the correct amount of slack in the lead: during inspiration the angle between the two limbs of the J should not exceed 80 degrees.

MEASUREMENT OF STIMULATION AND SENSING THRESHOLDS

Low stimulation and sensing thresholds are essential for satisfactory long-term pacing. High thresholds suggest that the cathode is not in close apposition to excitable tissue. Thresholds rise after pacemaker implantation, usually peaking 3 weeks to 3 months after surgery. If they become high, they may exceed the stimulation and sensing capabilities of the pulse generator. Thresholds are usually measured with a commercially produced pacing systems analyser. It is preferable to match the analyser with the generator to be implanted so that they have similar impulse generating and sensing circuits. The same unipolar or bipolar electrode configuration should be used as is planned to use with the implanted system.

Stimulation threshold

The stimulation threshold is the smallest electrical stimulus (delivered by the cathode outside the ventricular effective and relative refractory periods) which will consistently activate the myocardium.

To measure the stimulation threshold, the analyser is set to deliver impulses at 70 beats/min (or if there is no bradycardia at the time, 10 beats/min in excess of the spontaneous rate) with an impulse duration similar to that which the implanted pulse generator will deliver (often 0.5 ms) and a voltage output of 5 V. The threshold is then established by progressively reducing the output until failure of capture occurs; if the patient has no spontaneous rhythm, pacemaker output will have to be promptly increased to avoid asystole. At a pulse duration of 0.5 ms, a voltage threshold of less than 1 V is satisfactory: usually the threshold will be less than 0.5 V. Note that if the stimulation threshold is measured by progressively increasing the output from a subthreshold level it will be found to be higher: the Wedensky phenomenon.

It is important that the distal and proximal poles of the electrode are connected to the pacemaker cathode ( ) and anode (+), respectively. If the poles are reversed, the stimulation threshold will be substantially higher. The longer the duration of the pacing stimulus, the more energy is delivered and hence the lower is the stimulation threshold. However, the relationship is not linear: the range of efficient impulse duration, in terms of energy consumption, is 0.25–1.0 ms.

Sensing threshold

To ensure satisfactory sensing, it is important that the intracardiac electrogram resulting from spontaneous activity of the cardiac chamber to be paced is of sufficient amplitude. It is usually measured with a pacing systems analyser. Ventricular and atrial electrograms should be greater than 4 mV and 2 mV, respectively. In 'borderline' cases, the slew rate, i.e. the rate of change of signal voltage, is also important: low rates may result in failure to sense.

Lead impedance

The pacing systems analyser can also be used to measure lead impedance which is a measure of resistance to flow of current in the lead. It varies with lead type but is usually in the order of 400–800 ohms.

A low impedance suggests a break in insulation and hence leakage of current, whereas a high impedance points to lead fracture.

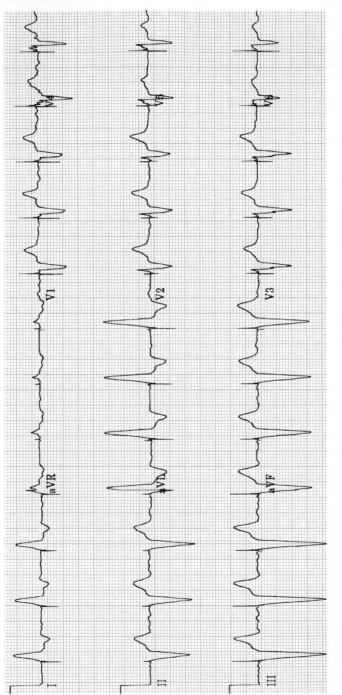

Figure 24.15 Right ventricular apical pacing: left axis deviation and left bundle branch block configuration

Paced ventricular electrogram

Pacing the right ventricular apex will lead to a ventricular complex with left axis deviation and left bundle branch block configuration (Figure 24.15). Right ventricular outflow tract pacing results in right axis deviation and left bundle branch block configuration (Figure 24.16) as would occur with right ventricular outflow tract tachycardia (see chapter 12). Inadvertent pacing of the left ventricle via a patent foramen ovale leads to a paced complex with right bundle branch block configuration.

Biventricular pacing for resynchronisation therapy typically results in a relatively narrow ventricular complex (Figure 24.17).

COMPLICATIONS OF PACEMAKER IMPLANTATION

Mild bruising is not uncommon but, occasionally, poor haemostasis will result in a haematoma which, if tense, should be evacuated.

Infection should occur in less than 1% of implantations and is virtually always staphyloccocal. Unless it is only superficial, explantation will usually be required even if antibiotics appear to help initially Ideally, the pacing lead(s) should be removed and this is essential if there has been systemic infection. It is usually easy to remove leads within the first few months of implantation by moderate sustained traction. However, removal late after implantation can be difficult, particularly if the leads have a passive fixation device such as fins. Use of special lead extraction devices such as 'locking stylettes' are often effective and reduce the risk of cardiac tamponade. Rarely, it is necessary to resort to thoracotomy. Alternatively, the lead can be shortened so that it no longer lies in the infected area, capping its proximal end and fixing it with a suture, but there is a risk of persistent infection and bacteraemia.

Several studies have shown that antibiotic cover, usually with flucloxacillin, reduces the risk of infection.

Erosion is a late complication but is often a consequence of implantation technique. Factors that predispose to erosion include creation of a pacemaker pocket which is too tight or too superficial, a very thin patient, and use of a generator with sharp corners. The skin will be found to be thinned around the site of erosion. Infection is often present but it is secondary to erosion. If the skin is broken, explantation will be necessary. Thinned reddened skin over the generator is a sign of 'threatened' erosion: the generator should be resited.

Lead displacement was once a common problem but with modern leads it occurs in less than 1% of implantations; it necessitates reoperation.

Complications of attempted subclavian vein puncture are infrequent. They include pneumothorax, haemothorax, air embolism, brachial plexus damage and puncture of the subclavian artery.

Fashioning of a generator pocket which is too large may allow spontaneous or intentional repeated rotation of the pulse generator which can cause dislodgement or fracture of the pacing lead: the 'twiddler's syndrome'.

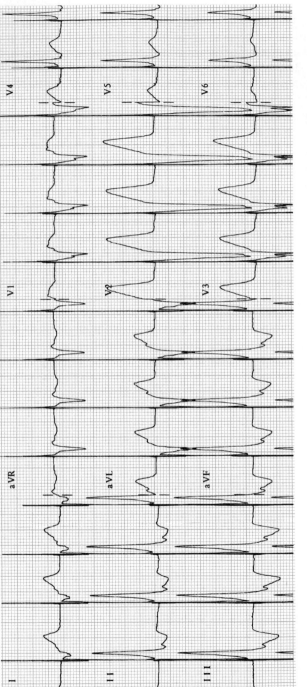

Figure 24.16 Right ventricular outflow tract pacing; right axis deviation and left bundle branch block configuration

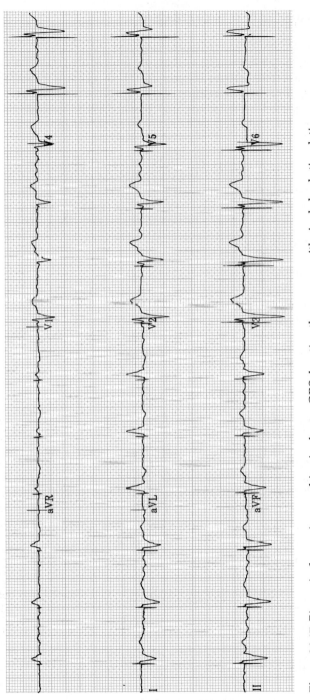

Figure 24.17 Biventricular pacing resulting in shorter QRS duration than occurs with single lead stimulation

COMPLICATIONS RELATED TO PULSE GENERATOR

Electromyographic interference

This common problem is virtually confined to unipolar pacing systems. Myopotentials generated from the underlying muscle are sensed by the pacemaker as spontaneous cardiac activity (Figure 24.18). In systems where sensed events inhibit output, inappropriate cessation of pacing will occur. Short periods of electromyographic inhibition are common and usually asymptomatic. Longer periods may cause syncope and necessitate adjustment to sensitivity, pacing mode or polarity.

Susceptibility to electromyographic inhibition can be demonstrated by asking the patient to extend his or her arms and then press his or her hands firmly together. Inhibition is only significant if it lasts for several seconds, particularly if the patient's symptoms are reproduced.

Muscle stimulation

This complication is also related to unipolar pacing. It is a consequence of the pacemaker can being the anode: stimulation of the underlying pectoral muscle occurs.

Generator failure

Premature generator failure does occur occasionally.

COMPLICATIONS RELATED TO PACING LEAD

Exit block

The development of excessive fibrous tissue, which is nonexcitable, around the cathode may increase the stimulation threshold to a level higher than the pacemaker's output. The result will be intermittent or persistent failure to pace without evidence of lead displacement (Figure 24.19). Exit block is most likely to occur in the first 3 weeks to 3 months after implantation when stimulation threshold is at its highest. Sometimes exit block is transient, otherwise lead repositioning will be required unless generator output can be increased by reprogramming (see below). Modern leads with low surface area, porous surfaced electrodes and positive fixation devices rarely give rise to this complication.

Lead fracture

With modern leads, fracture is rare. If it does occur it is usually at the point where the lead enters the venous system, at the site of a fixation suture or wherever there is excessive angulation of the lead. Lead fracture will cause intermittent or persistent failure to pace and sense. Lead impedance will be markedly elevated. Lead fracture can often be detected radiographically but should not be confused

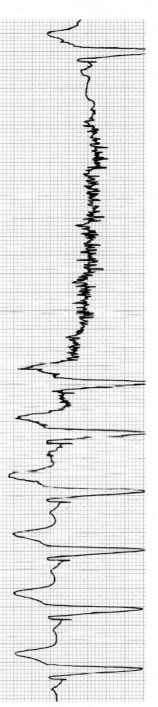

Figure 24.18 Electromyographic inhibition of a DDD pacemaker. Activities such as washing hands caused near-syncope. Corrected by decreasing pacemaker sensitivity

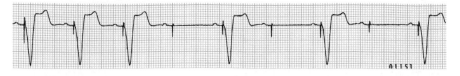

Figure 24.19 After three paced ventricular beats, there is intermittent exit block: pacing stimuli are not followed by ventricular complexes

with 'pseudofracture': the pressure of a tight ligature directly applied to the lead may compress the insulation and spread the coils of wire inside without interfering with lead function.

Insulation breakdown

This will allow leakage of current, which may cause stimulation of adjacent muscles, and hence premature battery depletion. Lead impedance will be markedly reduced. A tight ligature anchoring the lead without use of a rubber sleeve is the commonest cause. Some types of polyurethane insulation are prone to this problem.

Phrenic nerve and diaphragmatic stimulation

The phrenic nerve or diaphragm can sometimes be stimulated through the intervening thin myocardial walls by atrial and ventricular leads, respectively. Lead repositioning will be required unless, in programmable pacemakers, cessation of extracardiac stimulation can be achieved by output reduction.

Venous thrombosis

Clinically apparent subclavian vein thrombosis is rare and pulmonary embolism even rarer. Anticoagulant therapy is indicated. Angiographic studies have reported that asymptomatic venous thrombosis is not infrequent.

PACEMAKER PROGRAMMABILITY

A programmable pacemaker can be noninvasively adjusted in one or more of its functions by radiofrequency signals emitted from an external programming device. Programmability enables achievement of optimal pacemaker function for the individual patient and can also be used in the diagnosis and treatment of certain pacemaker complications; it reduces the need for pacemaker reoperation.

Simple programmable pacemakers permit alteration to rate and output. In multi-programmable pacemakers a wide variety of parameters can be adjusted. These are listed below together with typical options:

1. lower rate limit (30–150 beats/min);
2. output (2.5–7.5 V);

3. pulse duration (0.1–1.0 ms);
4. sensitivity (0.5–8 mV);
5. pacing mode (e.g. inhibited, triggered or rate response);
6. refractory period (200–500 ms);
7. pacing polarity (unipolar or bipolar);
8. AV delay (0–250 ms) (for dual-chamber pacemakers);
9. upper rate limits (100–180 beats/min) (for dual-chamber and rate-response pacemakers).

Some pacemakers are software based. Many functions are controlled by a micro-computer within the pacemaker which can be externally programmed. Functions can be modified and new developments incorporated that had not even been anticipated at the time of implantation.

Some examples of the advantages of programmability are discussed below.

In patients who are mainly in sinus rhythm, reduction of the stand-by rate will allow sinus rhythm to be maintained for longer periods and will therefore help to avoid the haemodynamic disadvantages of ventricular pacing. Reduction of stimulation rate may occasionally help in the management of angina. Sometimes an increase in rate is helpful in the treatment of cardiac failure or arrhythmias.

Usually, the stimulation threshold is a lot lower than the maximum output of a pacemaker; a reduction in output will prolong battery life. At regular intervals, the threshold can be measured by progressive reduction in output and then the output programmed to the threshold value plus a safety margin. Extracardiac stimulation can often be stopped by reduction in output without approaching the threshold level. Some pacemakers have a high output facility (e.g. ability to increase output from 5 to 10 V); use of this may avoid the need for reoperation should exit block, which may be a temporary problem, occur.

Increase in sensitivity of the amplifier circuits may help with undersensing, whereas inappropriate sensing of T waves or after-potentials may be dealt with by reduction in sensitivity or prolongation of refractory period.

Reduction in sensitivity may prevent electromyographic inhibition. Alternatively, reprogramming from inhibited to triggered mode will at least prevent bradycardia even if the electromyographic potentials reset the stimulation cycle. Another solution, which may also help with extracardiac stimulation, is to change from unipolar to bipolar pacing in systems that have this facility.

Atrial pacemakers require a higher sensitivity, because the atrial electrogram is usually of lower amplitude than its ventricular counterpart, and a longer refractory period to avoid sensing the far-field ventricular electrogram. A multiprogrammable generator can be adjusted for use as either an atrial or ventricular pacemaker.

In dual-chamber pacing systems, prolongation of the atrial refractory period may prevent endless loop tachycardia. Sometimes endless loop tachycardia can be prevented by reducing sensitivity of the atrial channel so that the atrial electrogram during sinus rhythm is sensed but the atrial electrogram resulting from retrograde conduction, which is usually of lower amplitude, is not detected. In patients with sick sinus syndrome, reprogramming from DDD to DDI or DVI modes will prevent endless loop tachycardia. Alteration from DDD to VVI may be required should atrial fibrillation develop.

Many pacemakers have the facility to program rate hysteresis. The interval after a sensed event which would trigger delivery of a pacemaker stimulus can be greater than the interval between paced beats. For example, a pacemaker can be programmed to stimulate the heart at 70 beats/min only if the spontaneous rate falls below 40 beats/min, thus helping to avoid problems which might occur with loss of AV synchrony.

PACEMAKER CLINIC

Patients with implanted pacemakers should regularly attend a follow-up clinic. The purposes are: to check that the pacemaker is working satisfactorily; to ensure that there are no pacing complications; to detect impending battery depletion so that generator replacement can be carried out before the patient is at risk; and to maintain a record of patients' locations should a recall of a particular generator or lead be necessary.

There are several indicators of impending battery depletion. First, a reduction in the stimulation rate which has to be measured precisely during fixed rate pacing usually initiated by placing a magnet over the pacemaker. Each type of pacemaker

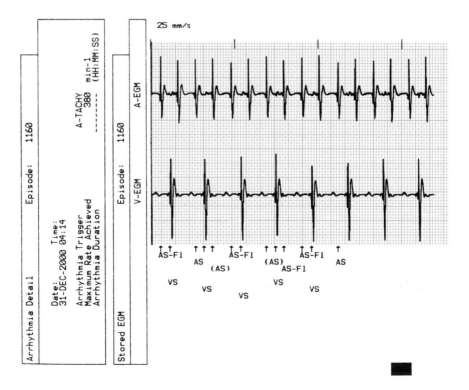

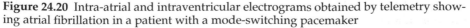

Figure 24.20 Intra-atrial and intraventricular electrograms obtained by telemetry showing atrial fibrillation in a patient with a mode-switching pacemaker

has its own characteristic 'end of life rate'; it is usually in the order of a 5–10% reduction of the 'beginning of life' rate. Most pulse generators have the facility to transmit data to the programmer, i.e. telemetry. Information about how the pacemaker has been programmed, battery status, stimulation and sensing thresholds, lead and battery impedance, patient details and intracardiac electrograms can be obtained (Figure 24.20). Marked reduction in battery voltage and increase in battery internal resistance are indicators of imminent battery depletion.

ELECTROMAGNETIC INTERFERENCE

External electromagnetic interference may affect pacemakers and cause either inhibition or reversion to the fixed rate mode, reprogramming or damage to the pacemaker circuitry. The many sources include electric motors in household devices, internal combustion engines, microwave ovens, radio transmitters, theft and weapon detection systems, arc-welding apparatus and radar. In practice, because pacemakers are well shielded and because of the use of appropriate filters, very few problems are encountered and patients should be reassured that the risks are minimal.

Clearly, if a patient feels dizzy near electrical equipment they should quickly walk away from it. If a patient's work brings him or her into close proximity with strong sources of electromagnetic interference, a bipolar pacemaker should be implanted.

ELECTRONIC ARTICLE SURVEILLANCE SYSTEMS (EAS) AND METAL DETECTORS

These could transiently inhibit or possibly reprogram a pacemaker. However, there are only a few reports of adverse incidents and no patient has been harmed. Current advice to patients is as follows.

1. Do not stay near an EAS system or metal detector longer than is necessary and do not lean against the system. It is sufficient to pass the system at an ordinary pace.
2. Be aware that EAS systems may be hidden or camouflaged in entrances and exits in many commercial establishments.
3. If scanning with a hand-held metal detector is necessary, warn the security personnel that you have an electronic medical device and ask them not to hold the metal detector near the device any longer than is absolutely necessary; or you may wish to ask for an alternative form of personal search.

MAGNETS

A magnet held directly over a pacemaker can activate its reed-switch and thereby function in a fixed rate mode. The effect should only last as long as the magnet is applied. Patients should be advised to avoid clothing and accessories which contain magnets.

CARDIOVERSION AND DEFIBRILLATION

Pacemaker damage can be prevented if the paddles are at least 15 cm from the generator and preferably are positioned so they are at right angles to the pacing system. Pacemaker function should be checked after the procedure.

DIATHERMY

Diathermy may damage a pacemaker, cause inappropriate inhibition or possibly precipitate ventricular fibrillation. If possible, a bipolar system should be used. If a unipolar system has to be used, output should be kept as low as possible. The active electrode should be kept at least 15 cm from the generator and the indifferent electrode sited as far away as possible so that its dipole is perpendicular to the pacing system. The pulse should be monitored so that diathermy could be interrupted if prolonged inhibition occurred. Ideally, the pacemaker should be checked prior to surgery. Some pacemakers are more prone to external interference when the batteries are approaching end of life. A pacemaker check should be performed soon after surgery.

RADIATION

Radiation for diagnostic purposes will not affect a pacemaker but therapeutic levels may cause damage. The pacemaker should be shielded and, if this is not possible, resiting of the generator should be considered.

MAGNETIC RESONANCE IMAGING

Limited experience with magnetic resonance imaging indicates that all pacemakers will revert to fixed-rate mode and some will pace at a dangerously fast rate. Pacemaker patients should not undergo magnetic resonance imaging.

LITHOTRIPSY

Shocks should not be focused directly over the pacemaker. The pacemaker should be programmed to non-rate-responsive VVI mode.

ELECTROCONVULSIVE THERAPY

Electroconvulsive therapy is safe.

Transcutaneous Electrical Nerve Stimulation (tens)

Unipolar pacemakers can be inhibited and it is recommended that the heart rhythm is monitored during initial TENS application in patients with bipolar systems.

Cellular phones

Mobile telephones may transiently interfere with pacemaker function. It is recommended that a mobile telephone is kept at least 15 cm from the pacemaker and when the 'phone is in use to use the ear opposite to the implant site.

DRIVING

In the United Kingdom, driving must cease if a patient has sino-atrial disease or atrioventricular block, and the arrhythmia has caused or is likely to cause incapacity. Patients may resume driving ordinary motor cars and motor cycles 1 week after implantation of a pacemaker provided there is no other disqualifying condition. Heavy goods and public service vehicle drivers are disqualified from driving for 6 weeks after pacemaker implantation. Licensing may be permitted thereafter provided there is no other disqualifying condition.

DIVING

The increased hydrostatic pressure underwater can compress pacemaker cans and cause device failure. Many pacemakers are affected at depths of 11 m. Manufacturers' advice should be sought.

CREMATION

A pacemaker must be explanted before cremation to avoid explosion.

Main points

- Long-term pacing is indicated in cases of symptomatic bradycardia and should also be considered in asymptomatic patients with second- or third-degree AV block or long pauses in sinus node activity.

- Ventricular demand pacing prevents normal AV synchrony and does not permit a chronotropic response to exercise.

- Loss of normal AV synchrony during ventricular demand pacing may cause symptomatic hypotension (pacemaker syndrome) and can be prevented by atrial or AV sequential pacing.

- Absence of a chronotropic response to exercise can markedly reduce exercise tolerance. Atrial synchronized ventricular pacing and rate-response systems sensitive to physiological parameters such as vibration, QT interval and respiration can facilitate a chronotropic response to exercise.

- The modern pacemaker is small, reliable and has a long battery life. Pacemaker infection is the commonest reason for reoperation. Many other complications can be resolved without operation if the pacemaker is programmable.

CHAPTER 25

Automatic implantable cardiovertor defibrillator

Sudden cardiac death due to ventricular fibrillation or tachycardia is common. Anti-arrhythmic drugs do not significantly reduce mortality. The automatic cardiovertor defibrillator is an implantable device which can recognize and automatically terminate these arrhythmias by delivering an appropriate electrical therapy.

The three therapies are:

1. precisely timed pacing stimuli to terminate ventricular tachycardia (*see* Figure 12.13);
2. low-energy (0.5–10 J) DC shock to terminate ventricular tchycardia, i.e. cardioversion (Figure 25.1);
3. higher energy (15–34 J) DC shock to terminate ventricular tachycardia or fibrillation, i.e. defibrillation (Figure 25.2).

In addition, the device can act as a pacemaker to prevent bradycardia.

The first defibrillator was implanted in 1980. Since then there have been great strides in technology. Early devices were very large, necessitating implantation in the rectus sheath, and employed epicardial leads. Newer devices are somewhat larger than a pacemaker and can be implanted subcutaneously, over the pectoral muscles. Only a single transvenous lead, introduced via the cephalic or subclavian vein, is required: the can of the device acts as an indifferent electrode. Shocks are delivered between the can and one or, in some cases, two coils on the lead. Devices last approximately 8 years.

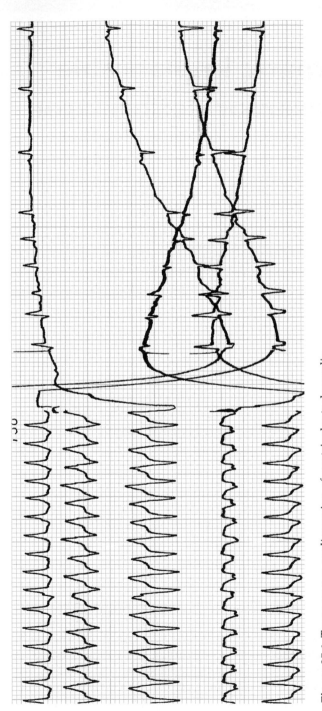

Figure 25.1 Transvenous cardioversion of ventricular tachycardia

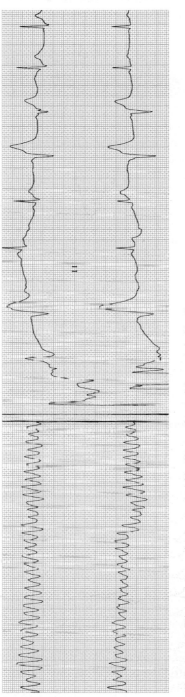

Figure 25.2 Termination of ventricular fibrillation by implanted defibrillator

Implantation is usually carried out under local anaesthesia. Intravenous sedation is given prior to defibrillation testing: it is necessary to induce fibrillation at least twice to ensure a satisfactory defibrillation threshold – usually less than 18 J (Figure 25.3).

INDICATIONS

Many patients with cardiac disease are at risk of sudden death due to ventricular tachycardia or fibrillation and might benefit from the device. However, its benefits have to be weighed against its shortcomings, as discussed below.

SECONDARY PREVENTION

Secondary prevention is therapy to deal with a recurrence of ventricular tachycardia or fibrillation. In accordance with current United Kingdom guidelines, defibrillator implantation should be considered for patients who present with the following, provided the arrhythmia is not due to acute myocardial infarction and there is no correctable cause:

1. survivors of sudden cardiac death caused by ventricular fibrillation or tachycardia;
2. spontaneous sustained ventricular tachycardia causing syncope or significant haemodynamic compromise;
3. sustained ventricular tachycardia without syncope or cardiac arrest in patients who have a left ventricular ejection fraction less than 35% but are no worse than class 3 of the New York Heart Association functional classification of heart failure.

Several major clinical trials have demonstrated that, in the above groups of patients, the automatic cardiovertor defibrillator reduces mortality as compared with anti-arrhythmic drug therapy.

PRIMARY PREVENTION

Primary prevention is therapy for patients who are at high risk of death or collapse from ventricular tachycardia or fibrillation who have not yet sustained these arrhythmias. In accordance with current United Kingdom guidelines, defibrillator implantation should be considered for patients with the following.

1. Previous myocardial infarction and all of the following:
   (i) nonsustained ventricular tachycardia on ambulatory electrocardiography;
   (ii) inducible ventricular tachycardia at electrophysiological testing;
   (iii) left ventricular ejection fraction of less than 35% and with symptoms no worse than class III of the New York Heart Association.

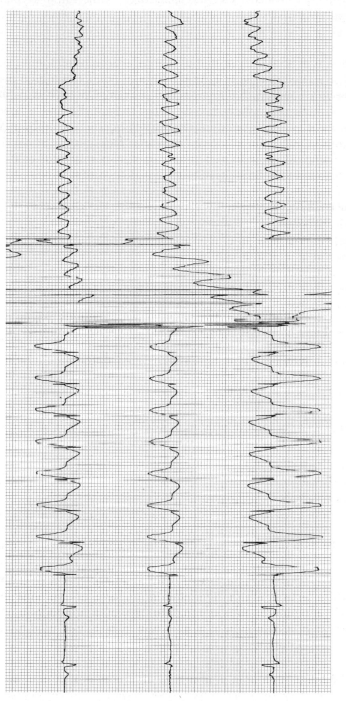

Figure 25.3 Initiation of ventricular fibrillation by delivering a low-energy DC shock on the T wave of the eighth paced beat

These recommendations are based on two studies that have shown that mortality in patients with the above characteristics is reduced by the automatic cardiovertor defibrillator as compared with anti-arrhythmic drug therapy, mainly amiodarone.

However, since thrombolysis for acute myocardial infarction has become widespread practice, several studies have shown that nonsustained ventricular tachycardia (which was defined in these studies as three or more ventricular ectopic beats in succession at a rate in excess of 120 beats/min) is not in fact a good predictor of sudden death in patients with a low ejection fraction. Only 3% of patients were found to have both nonsustained ventricular tachycardia and a low ejection fraction. Further studies in patients with poor left ventricular function are under way. It is possible that inducibility of ventricular tachycardia irrespective of the presence or absence of nonsustained ventricular tachycardia plus or minus other factors may be found to be better predictors of sudden cardiac death.

2. A cardiac condition in which it is recognized that the patient is at high risk of sudden death including:
    (i) long QT syndrome;
    (ii) hypertrophic cardiomyopathy;
    (iii) Brugada syndrome;
    (iv) arrhythmogenic right ventricular dysplasia;
    (iv) following repair of tetralogy of Fallot.

In terms of primary prevention, one of the main indications of high risk in conditions (i)–(iv) is a family history of premature, sudden cardiac death. Following repair of Fallot's tetralogy, prolonged QRS duration has been shown to be a predictor of sudden death.

DEFIBRILLATOR FUNCTION

TIERED THERAPY

Some ventricular tachycardias can be terminated by 'anti-tachycardia pacing', i.e. delivery of 6–10 ventricular stimuli in rapid succession (*see* Figure 12.13). Ventricular fibrillation can only be terminated by delivery of a high-energy shock. The advantages of terminating ventricular tachycardia by anti-tachycardia pacing are that it is painless and battery energy is conserved. However, anti-tachycardia pacing is not only sometimes ineffective but may cause acceleration of the tachycardia.

Detection of ventricular tachycardia and fibrillation is based mainly on the rate of sensed ventricular electrograms. Usually, rate criteria are used to place the arrhythmia in one of three zones listed below.

Slow VT zone

Ventricular tachycardia at a rate of 140–160 beats/min is termed 'slow'. There is a fairly high chance that anti-tachycardia pacing will be effective. It is usual to program the device to attempt to terminate the tachycardia several times before proceeding to cardioversion, i.e. delivering a synchronized 5–10 J shock. Either 'burst' or 'ramp' pacing can be used. With the former, the interval between stimuli is constant, whereas with the latter, the interval between successive stimuli is decreased by approximately 8–10 ms. For most patients, burst and ramp pacing are in fact equally effective. Initial attempts at pacing typically employ a train of 6–8 impulses at 81–84% of the tachycardia cycle length. If ineffective, the device will then deliver more aggressive therapies, e.g. 8–10 impulses with shorter cycle lengths; 78–81% of tachycardia cycle length.

It is important to ensure that the lower limit of the range of tachycardia detection does not overlap with a heart rate that the patient is likely to achieve during sinus rhythm, otherwise the device will deliver therapy inappropriately.

Fast VT zone

'Fast ventricular tachycardia' is usually defined as a rate between 160 and 190 beats/min. There is only a modest chance that it can be terminated by pacing and often little time can be allowed for pacing because it is likely that a tachycardia in this range will cause collapse. It is usual to program the device to attempt anti-tachycardia pacing up to three times. If unsuccessful, the device will then proceed to deliver a 10-J shock and, if necessary, a shock at maximum energy.

VF zone

A rate in excess of 190 beats/min is assumed to be ventricular fibrillation. Electrograms during ventricular fibrillation are of low amplitude. To avoid failure to detect ventricular fibrillation, only 80% of sensed electrograms over a period of approximately 6 s are required to meet the rate criteria: ventricular fibrillation is assumed and a high-energy shock (18–34 J) will be discharged after a further 6 s. If fibrillation is redetected, further shocks will be delivered.

ELECTROGRAM RECORDING

Current implantable defibrillators can store electrocardiograms prior to and immediately after the device has initiated anti-tachycardia pacing or has delivered a shock. Thus it is possible to ensure that appropriate therapy was initiated and that the device had not responded to a supraventricular tachycardia (Figure 25.4).

DUAL-CHAMBER AUTOMATIC CARDIOVERTOR DEFIBRILLATORS

Devices are now available which facilitate atrial pacing and sensing. Clearly, an atrial lead is required. Dual-chamber devices provide the same benefits as dual-chamber pacemakers for the management of bradycardia. In addition, atrial sensing enables better discrimination between supraventricular and ventricular arrhythmias (Figures 25.5–25.7).

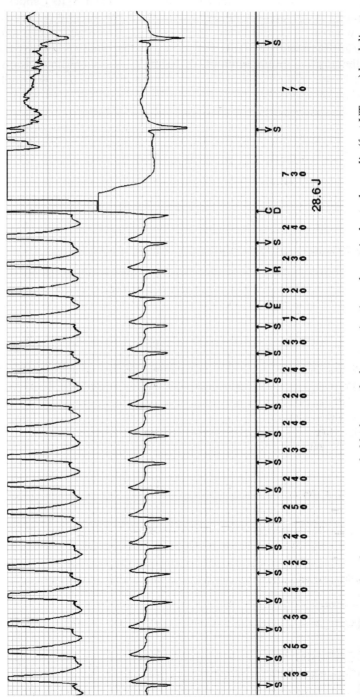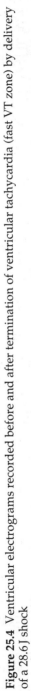

Figure 25.4 Ventricular electrograms recorded before and after termination of ventricular tachycardia (fast VT zone) by delivery of a 28.6 J shock

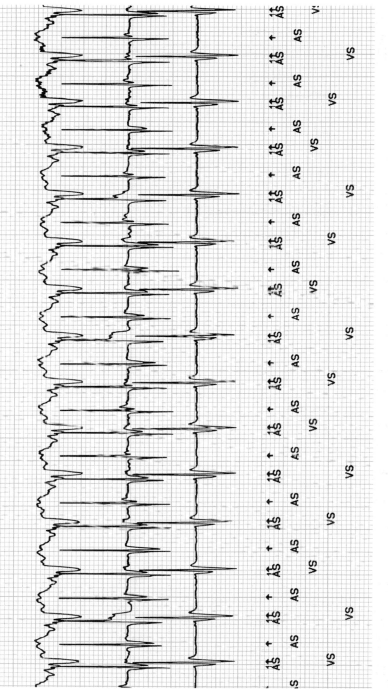

Figure 25.5 Intra-atrial (middle trace) and intraventricular electrograms (lower trace) recorded during tachycardia show that atrial rate exceeded ventricular rate pointing to atrial arrhythmia

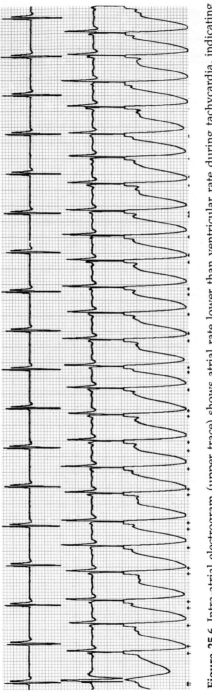
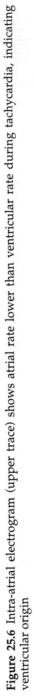

Figure 25.6 Intra-atrial electrogram (upper trace) shows atrial rate lower than ventricular rate during tachycardia, indicating ventricular origin

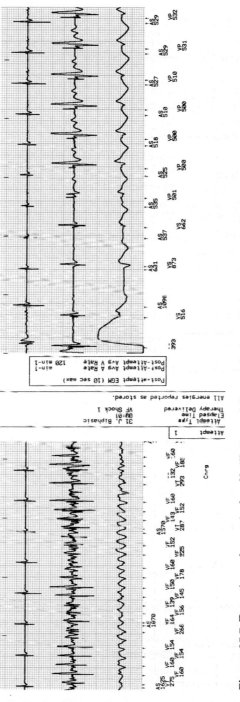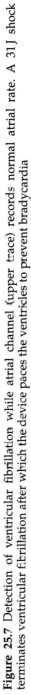

Figure 25.7 Detection of ventricular fibrillation while atrial channel (upper trace) records normal atrial rate. A 31J shock terminates ventricular fibrillation after which the device paces the ventricles to prevent bradycardia

LIMITATIONS

Discharge of a high-energy DC shock in a conscious patient results in sudden marked chest discomfort and may cause considerable distress! Patients describe experiencing sensations such as 'a blow to the chest' or 'a spasm making the whole body jump'.

The device is not suitable for patients with frequently recurrent or incessant arrhythmias, since it would be activated too often.

Inappropriate discharge may occur in response to a rapid ventricular rate during atrial fibrillation or other supraventricular tachycardia.

An implantable defibrillator is often regarded as an alternative to anti-arrhythmic drugs. However, to almost lose consciousness from ventricular fibrillation and then be defibrillated is not a pleasant experience. Ideally, the implantable defibrillator should act as a 'back-up' device. Often, anti-arrhythmic drugs, usually amiodarone or sotalol, are required to reduce the frequency of ventricular arrhythmias requiring shock delivery or to prevent supraventricular arrhythmias. It should be noted that amiodarone may raise the 'defibrillation threshold' and possibly render the device ineffective, if the threshold was already high.

Many patients benefit psychologically from the peace of mind that the potentially life-saving facility of an implantable defibrillator offers. However, some patients, particularly those who have received inappropriate or frequent shocks, dread further shocks and are psychologically disturbed as a consequence.

Currently, costs are high. In the United Kingdom, implantation costs are in excess of £15 000.

PRECAUTIONS

Implantable defibrillators are subject to electromagnetic interference in the same way as pacemakers, as discussed above. Application of a magnet over a defibrillator will inactivate it. Clothing and accessories containing magnets should not be worn.

A defibrillator must be inactivated during implantation or removal otherwise the operator may receive an electric shock.

DRIVING

Discharge of a defibrillator during motor vehicle driving will at very least cause distraction and will probably result in temporary incapacity. It may save the driver's life but could endanger others' lives. Furthermore, the device may be triggered by ventricular arrhythmias, which would not have caused collapse, and inappropriate discharge might result from supraventricular tachycardia or technical failure such as lead fracture.

Approaches to licensing drivers vary from country to country. Below are the regulations which apply in the United Kingdom.

In patients receiving a device for secondary prevention, driving may occur when the following criteria can be met.

1. The first device has been implanted for at least 6 months.
2. The device has not administered therapy (shock and/or symptomatic anti-tachycardia pacing) within the last 6/12 (except during formal clinical testing).
3. Any previous therapy following device implantation has not been accompanied by incapacity (whether caused by the device or arrhythmia) in the preceding 5 years, unless the underlying cause has been identified and controlled.
4. A period of 1 month off driving must occur following any revision of the device (generator and/or electrode) or alteration of anti-arrhythmic drug treatment.
5. The device is subject to regular review with interrogation.
6. There is no other disqualifying condition.

The licence shall be subject to annual review.

Permanent licence refusal or revocation is recommended for drivers of large lorries and buses (Group 2, LGV, PCV licence).

In patients receiving a device for primary prevention, i.e. if an automatic cardiovertor defibrillator has been implanted in an individual considered to be at high risk of significant arrhythmia as a result of relevant family history or other condition, but prior to implantation a significant arrhythmia has not occurred, then following implantation, driving must cease for 1 month and may recommence thereafter subject to satisfactory out-patient review at that time. The DVLA (Driver and Vehicle Licensing Agency) need not be notified. Should the device subsequently deliver anti-tachycardia pacing and/or shock therapy (except during formal clinical testing), then the usual criteria apply and the DVLA should be notified.

Main points

- The automatic cardiovertor defibrillator is an implantable device which can recognize and automatically terminate ventricular tachycardia or fibrillation by delivering precisely timed pacing stimuli or a DC shock. The device can also act as a pacemaker to prevent bradycardia.

- Implantation procedures for defibrillators and pacemakers are similar.

- Patients at high risk from a recurrence of ventricular tachycardia or fibrillation (secondary prevention) or at high risk from a condition which might cause death from ventricular tachycardia or fibrillation (primary prevention) are candidates for implantation of an automatic cardiovertor defibrillator.

CHAPTER 26

Radiofrequency catheter ablation

Radiofrequency catheter ablation has transformed the treatment of many rhythm disturbances, particularly those of supraventricular origin. For several arrhythmias it is not just another therapeutic option but a first-line treatment, offering a cure and obviating the need for anti-arrhythmic drugs with their associated unwanted effects. Success rates over 90% are being widely achieved. The risks are low. The purpose of this chapter is to illustrate briefly some of the main applications of radiofrequency catheter ablation.

The procedure is usually carried out under local anaesthesia, with or without sedation, in a cardiac catheterization laboratory. The sequence of cardiac activation during normal and abnormal rhythms is studied by recording electrograms from various intracardiac sites using multipolar catheter electrodes introduced via percutaneous puncture of the femoral vein and, if necessary, the femoral artery. The electrodes also facilitate introduction of pacing stimuli that can initiate and terminate tachycardias.

Mapping during normal and paced rhythms and during tachycardia enable location of the re-entrant circuit or focus causing the arrhythmia. Radiofrequency energy (which is high-frequency alternating current) is delivered via a special catheter electrode. This has a deflectable end, enabling the tip to be precisely positioned at the target site. Radiofrequency energy is delivered for 30–120 s. The endocardium in contact with the tip and the myocardium beneath is heated to 50–70ºC and is thereby coagulated. Surrounding myocardium is not damaged.

NORMAL SINUS RHYTHM

Figure 26.1 shows typical findings during normal sinus rhythm. Recordings are usually made at a paper speed of 100 mm/s. Below the six surface ECG leads are recordings from three intracardiac sites: high right atrium, tricuspid valve and the coronary sinus.

HIGH RIGHT ATRIAL ELECTROGRAM

An electrode positioned in the high right atrium is close to the sinus node. It records the earliest atrial activity during each cardiac cycle. It coincides with the onset of the P wave seen on the surface ECG.

HIS BUNDLE ELECTROGRAM

The His bundle electrogram is recorded by positioning an electrode across the tricuspid valve. The following three waves can be seen.

First, there is the A wave due to activation of the adjacent low right atrium.

Second is the H wave: the electrogram resulting from activation of the His bundle. The interval between A and H waves indicates the speed of conduction through the AV node.

The third wave is the V wave, which is the ventricular electrogram. It coincides with the QRS complex on the surface ECG. The H–V interval indicates the time of transmission by the His bundle and bundle branches from the AV node to the ventricular myocardium. Often, as in this example, electrograms are recorded from two pairs of electrodes on the multipolar catheter across the tricuspid valve, so proximal and distal His bundle electrograms can be obtained.

CORONARY SINUS ELECTROGRAMS

The coronary sinus runs in the groove between the left atrium and left ventricle. Activity from both the left atrium and left ventricle can be recorded.

A large left atrial electrogram can be seen, which is followed by a smaller wave resulting from left ventricular activity.

Mapping

The figure provides a simple example of how the path of an activating impulse can be 'mapped'. It shows how the atrial impulse originates in the high right atrium (i.e.

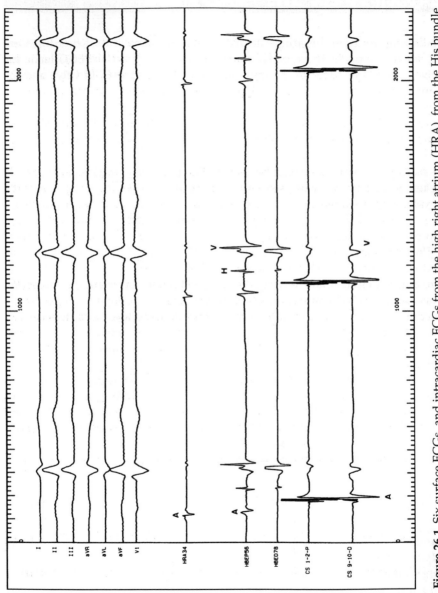

Figure 26.1 Six surface ECGs, and intracardiac ECGs from the high right atrium (HRA), from the His bundle (HBEP = proximal, HBED = distal) and coronary sinus (CS ... P = proximal; CS ... D = distal; A, H and V = atrial, His bundle and ventricular electrograms, respectively).

close to the sinus node), passes to the low right atrium, near to the AV node, and then to the left atrium as recorded by the coronary sinus electrodes.

WOLFF–PARKINSON–WHITE SYNDROME

The main way to locate an accessory pathway is to identify the site of earliest ventricular activation during sinus rhythm (or atrial pacing). An electrogram at this site will precede the onset of the delta wave in the surface ECG (Figure 26.2). Sometimes, it is possible to actually demonstrate an accessory pathway potential (Figure 26.3).

Figure 26.4 shows how the surface ECG and electrogram at the site of radiofrequency delivery change as the accessory pathway is ablated by radiofrequency energy.

Left-sided pathways are ablated by introducing a catheter into the left ventricle via the femoral artery (or by transseptal puncture) and positioning its tip across the mitral valve ring. Free right wall accessory pathways are ablated by introducing a catheter from the femoral vein and positioning across the tricuspid valve ring. Posteroseptal and anteroseptal pathways are also ablated by a catheter in the right heart. Posteroseptal pathways are found near the mouth of the coronary sinus. Anteroseptal pathways are located close to the bundle of His.

There is a small risk that anteroseptal and, to a much lesser extent, posteroseptal pathway ablation might cause complete heart block and need long-term pacing.

Sometimes, T wave memory following successful ablation causes unnecessary concern (Figure 26.5).

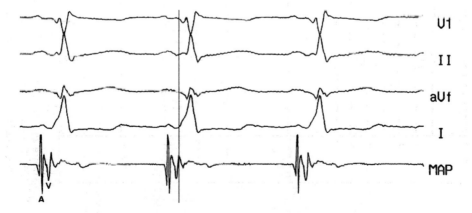

Figure 26.2 Wolff–Parkinson–White syndrome. The vertical line marks the onset of the delta wave on the surface ECG. The tip of the mapping electrode has been positioned at the site of successful ablation. Both A and V waves can be seen in the mapping electrogram. The V wave precedes the onset of the surface ECG delta wave by 25 ms.

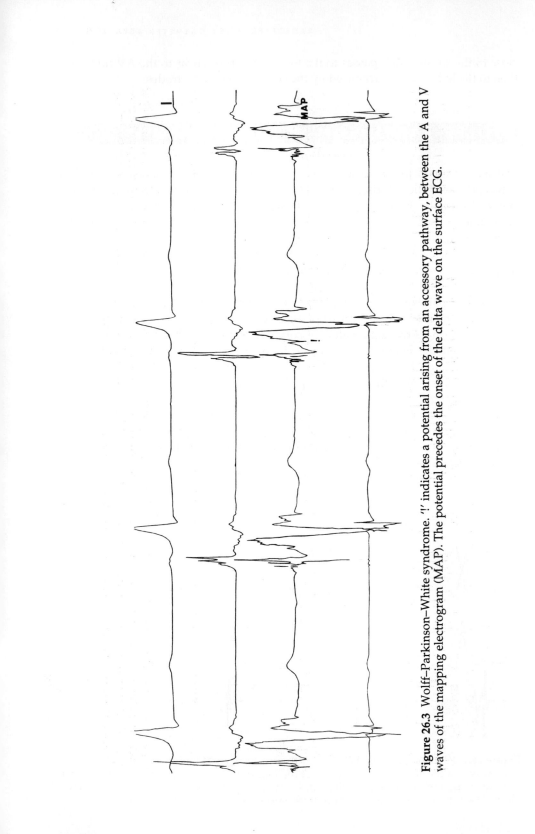

Figure 26.3 Wolff–Parkinson–White syndrome. '!' indicates a potential arising from an accessory pathway, between the A and V waves of the mapping electrogram (MAP). The potential precedes the onset of the delta wave on the surface ECG.

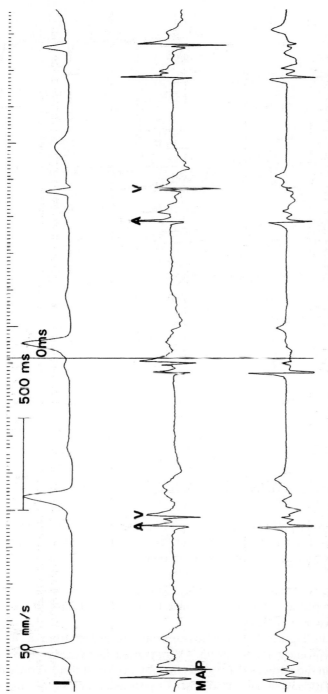

Figure 26.4 Wolff–Parkinson–White syndrome. Radiofrequency energy is delivered after the first three beats and interrupts accessory pathway conduction. The vertical line demonstrates that before ablation, ventricular activity in the mapping electrogram (MAP) precedes the onset of the surface ECG delta wave. After ablation, the delta wave disappears and ventricular activity in the mapping electrogram succeeds rather than precedes the surface ECG QRS complex

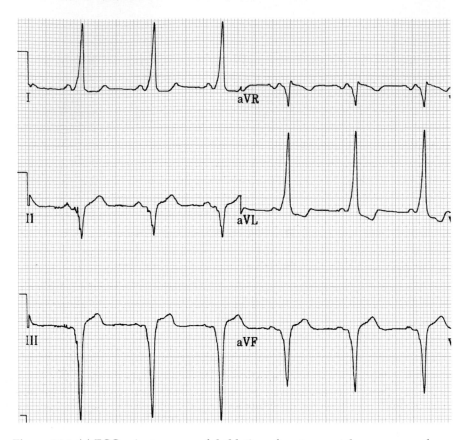

Figure 26.5 (a) ECG prior to successful ablation of posteroseptal accessory pathway

CONCEALED ACCESSORY PATHWAYS

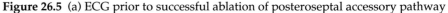

A concealed accessory pathway can transmit impulses from ventricles to atria and therefore facilitate atrioventricular re-entrant tachycardia, but cannot conduct from atria to ventricles and thus there will be no delta wave or PR shortening during sinus rhythm.

Concealed pathways have to be located during AV re-entrant tachycardia (or rapid ventricular pacing). The site of earliest atrial activation will indicate the location of the accessory pathway.

For example, in Figure 26.6 electrograms are recorded from a multipolar electrode in the coronary sinus during AV re-entrant tachycardia. Earliest atrial activity is found in the mid-coronary sinus thereby demonstrating a concealed left-sided free wall pathway. An electrode (MAP) positioned across the mitral valve close to CS 7,8 of the coronary sinus electrode showed even earlier atrial activity. Delivery of radiofrequency energy at that site blocked the accessory pathway.

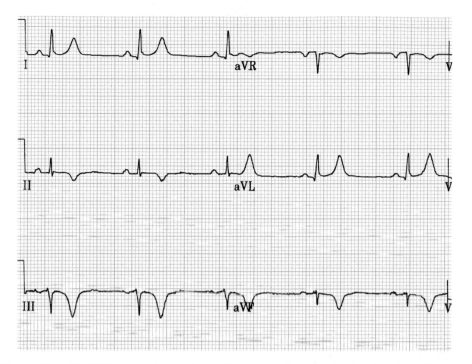

Figure 26.5 (b) ECG on next day showed absence of pre-excitation but deep T wave inversion in inferior leads caused concern about ischaemic damage. In fact it was due to 'T wave memory', i.e. the T wave continues in the same direction as the QRS complex in that lead prior to ablation. The ECG had returned to normal within 2 weeks.

ATRIOVENTRICULAR NODAL TACHYCARDIA

The hallmark of this arrhythmia is the very short conduction time from ventricles to atria during tachycardia (*see* chapter 9): atrial activity coincides with, or just precedes or just follows the ventricular complex. This is reflected in all intracardiac electrograms (Figure 26.7).

'Slow pathway ablation' is the most common approach to atrioventricular nodal re-entrant tachycardia. The slow pathway is one of the two limbs of the re-entrant. It is usually located just superior and anterior to the mouth of the coronary sinus. A typical slow pathway electrogram can be recorded (Figure 26.8). Radiofrequency energy delivered to the site at which this electrogram is obtained usually leads to a short period of junctional rhythm, after which the tachycardia can no longer be induced.

There is a 2–3% risk of causing complete heart block when attempting slow pathway ablation. This risk can be minimized by immediately interrupting delivery of radiofrequency energy, if a junctional tachycardia rather than junctional rhythm occurs or if there is loss of ventriculoatrial conduction during junctional rhythm. Patients should be informed of the small possibility that the procedure will lead to pacemaker implantation.

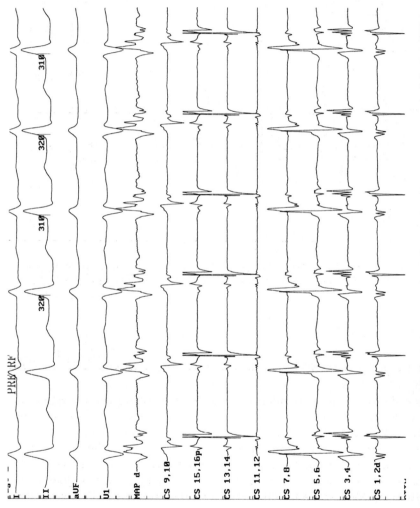

Figure 26.6 Concealed left-sided accessory AV pathway. The trace is recorded during AV re-entrant tachycardia. It shows four surface ECGs, electrograms from a mapping electrode (MAP) placed across the mitral valve, and a series of coronary sinus electrograms from proximal (CS 9,10) to distal positions (CS 1,2). The sequence of atrial electrograms in the coronary sinus indicates a left-sided free wall accessory pathway

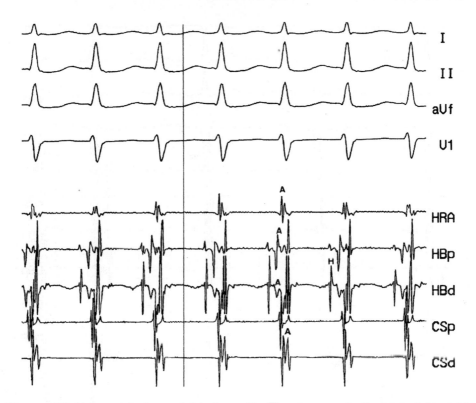

I

II

aVf

U1

A

HRA

A

HBp

H

HBd

CSp

A

CSd

Figure 26.7 Atrioventricular nodal tachycardia. The A waves in the high right atrial (HRA), His bundle (HB) and coronary sinus (CS) electrograms are almost coincident with ventricular activation. (The His bundle electrogram (H) precedes the A and V waves.)

ATRIAL FIBRILLATION AND FLUTTER

In some patients with these arrhythmias, anti-arrhythmic therapy is ineffective or cannot be tolerated. If uncontrolled, these arrhythmias cannot only cause unpleasant symptoms but sometimes also cardiac failure.

Radiofrequency energy can be used to ablate the AV node and thus protect the ventricles from the rapid atrial activity caused by these rhythm disturbances. AV node ablation will, of course, lead to complete heart block. In contrast to ablation for other arrhythmias, AV nodal ablation is palliative rather than curative, since the procedure necessitates pacemaker implantation.

Ablation of the AV node is usually easy and failure is rare. The ablating electrode is positioned across the tricuspid valve to record a large His bundle electrogram. The tip of the electrode is then withdrawn slightly in order to record a large A wave with a smaller H wave (Figure 26.9). Delivery of radiofrequency energy usually first causes a junctional tachycardia and then complete AV block (Figure 26.10).

Occasionally, it is not possible to ablate the AV node via the right heart. In these cases, a left-sided approach is usually successful. The ablating electrode can be

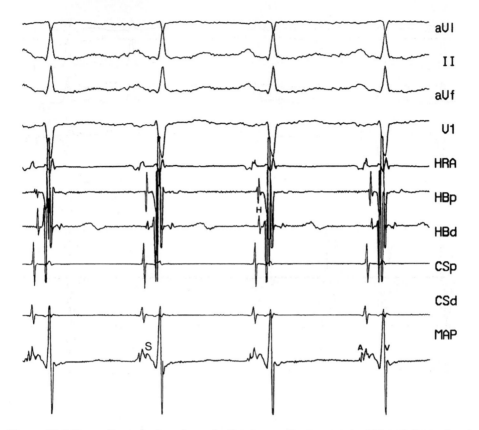

Figure 26.8 Recordings during sinus rhythm in a patient prone to AV nodal re-entrant tachycardia. The mapping electrode is positioned just superior and anterior to the mouth of the coronary sinus. A typical slow pathway electrogram (S) has been recorded: a small A wave followed by continuous electrical activity and then a large V wave

passed across the aortic valve into the left ventricle. A large His bundle electrogram can be easily found inferior to the aortic valve on the interventricular septum.

CARDIAC PACING

Choice of the most appropriate pacing mode is important. The pacemaker must provide a chronotropic response. A VVIR pacemaker should be used in persistent atrial fibrillation or flutter. In patients with paroxysmal atrial arrhythmias, a DDDR pacemaker, preferably with mode-switching facility is required (*see* chapter 16).

Patients who have developed ventricular dysfunction as a result of sustained high ventricular rates during atrial fibrillation are at a small risk of ventricular fibrillation within the first day after ablation. This risk can be minimized by pacing at ≥ 80 beats/min for the first couple of weeks after ablation.

There are advantages in implanting the pacemaker prior to AV node ablation. One can ensure that there are no pacemaker complications before committing the

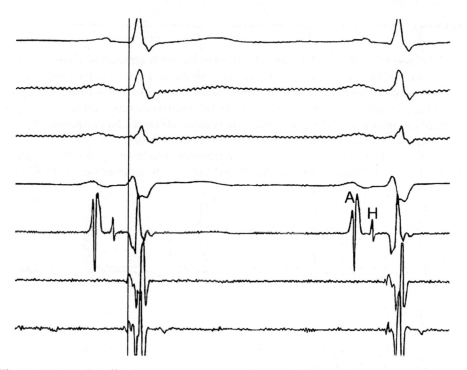

Figure 26.9 His bundle electrogram prior to AV nodal ablation showing large A wave and small H wave

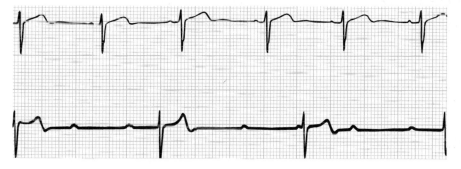

Figure 26.10 Patient with paroxysmal atrial fibrillation before (upper trace) and after (lower trace) AV node ablation

patient to the need of a pacemaker. Furthermore, in some patients with paroxysmal atrial fibrillation, it has been found that pacing (plus or minus an anti-arrhythmic drug) will prevent or markedly reduce the frequency of atrial fibrillation and thereby obviate the need for AV node ablation. Pacing the atrial septum appears to be more effective than pacing the atrial appendage.

ATRIAL FLUTTER

Atrial flutter is caused by a re-entrant circuit in the right atrium (*see* chapter 7). It is possible to ablate myocardium in this circuit and thereby prevent atrial flutter without the need for pacing. However, the success rate is currently lower than with other types of ablation and there is a significant recurrence rate. Furthermore, atrial fibrillation sometimes develops after successful ablation. Nevertheless, ablation compares favourably with medical treatment of atrial flutter.

The most effective method is to deliver a number of radiofrequency 'burns' along a line from the posterior part of the tricuspid valve to the inferior vena cava (Figure 26.11).

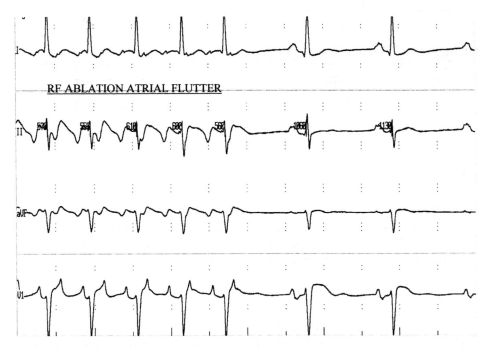

Figure 26.11 Leads I, II, aVF, V1 (100 mm/s) during atrial flutter as line of radiofrequency lesions between tricuspid valve and inferior vena cava is completed: sinus rhythm returns

RIGHT VENTRICULAR OUTFLOW TRACT TACHYCARDIA

The origin of this tachycardia is just below the pulmonary valve. It can be located by seeking the earliest site of ventricular activation (Figure 26.12) and by pace-mapping (Figure 26.13).

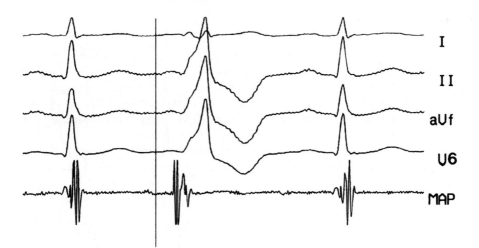

I

II

aVf

V6

MAP

Figure 26.12 The second beat is a ventricular ectopic beat arising from the site of origin of right ventricular outflow tract tachycardia. In contrast to the normal sinus beats before and after, the mapping electrode records ventricular activity earlier than seen on the surface ECGs.

FASCICULAR VENTRICULAR TACHYCARDIA

Fascicular tachycardia arises from the posterior fascicle, or rarely, anterior fascicle of the left bundle branch. The appropriate site for delivery of radiofrequency energy can be found by seeking the earliest area of left ventricular activation and is confirmed by the demonstration of a fascicular potential (Figures 26.14 and 26.15).

VENTRICULAR TACHYCARDIA DUE TO STRUCTURAL HEART DISEASE

Ablation of ventricular tachycardias due to myocardial infarction or cardiomyopathy is challenging. Success rates are lower and procedure times much longer than for ablation of other arrhythmias. Identification of the optimal ablation site is usually performed during tachycardia. Therefore, ablation can only usually be attempted in patients with slower, well tolerated tachycardias.

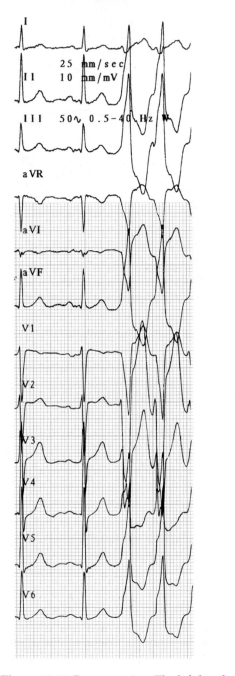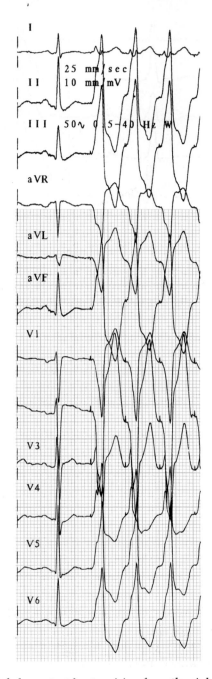

Figure 26.13 Pace mapping. The left-hand panel shows two beats arising from the right ventricular outflow tract. Pacing at a site just inferior to the pulmonary valve resulted in an almost identical configuration. Radiofrequency energy to this site abolished right ventricular outflow tract tachycardia

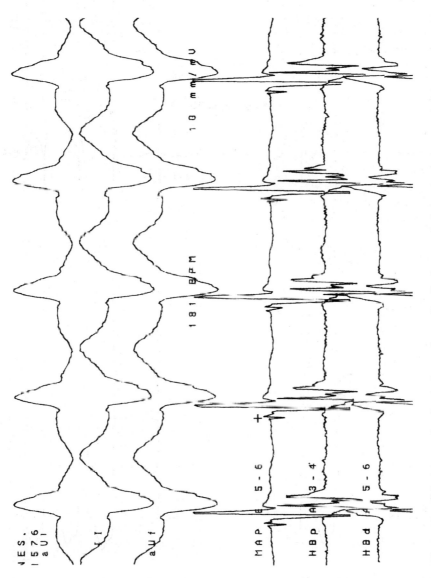

Figure 26.14 Left posterior fascicular tachycardia. Early ventricular activation preceded by a fascicular potential (+) is recorded at a site in the posteroapical portion of the left interventricular septum (MAP).

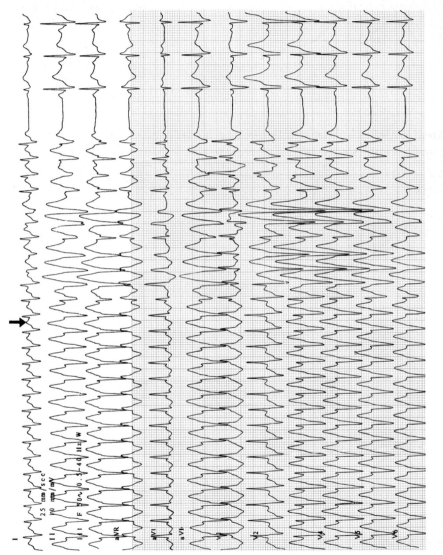

Figure 26.15 Left posterior fascicular tachycardia (25 mm/s). Delivery of radiofrequency energy (arrow) to the site demonstrated in Figure 26.14 quickly led to termination of tachycardia, which could then no longer be initiated

Main points

- Radiofrequency catheter ablation can be used to treat many cardiac arrhythmias and has become a first-line treatment for supraventricular tachycardias and ventricular tachycardias not caused by structural heart disease.

- An accessory pathway is located by seeking the earliest site of ventricular activation during sinus rhythm or the earliest site of atrial activation during AV re-entrant tachycardia.

- Atrioventricular nodal tachycardia is characterized by very short ventriculo-atrial conduction times as measured at all atrial sites. Delivery of radiofrequency energy to a site close to the coronary sinus os will ablate the slow AV nodal pathway.

- Atrial flutter can be treated by ablating the isthmus in the right atrial re-entrant circuit. Success rates compare favourably with medical therapy.

- AV nodal ablation is very effective in atrial fibrillation that cannot be controlled by medication. It necessitates pacemaker implantation.

- Fascicular and right ventricular outflow tract ventricular tachycardias can be cured by ablation.

CHAPTER 27

Arrhythmias for interpretation

Examples of a variety of arrhythmias are given. Their interpretations can be found at the end of the chapter.

As is often the case in practice, there may be more than one observation to make about each example.

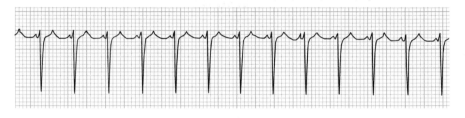

Figure 27.1

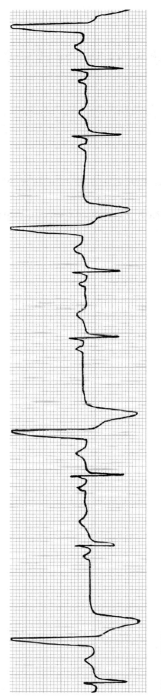

Figure 27.2

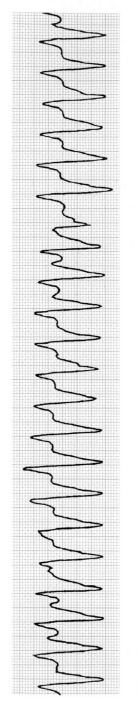

Figure 27.3

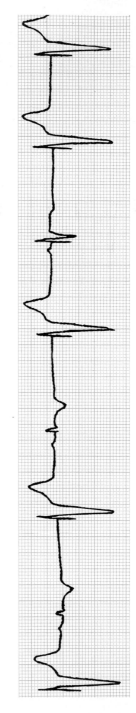

Figure 27.4

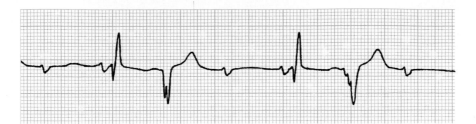

Figure 27.5

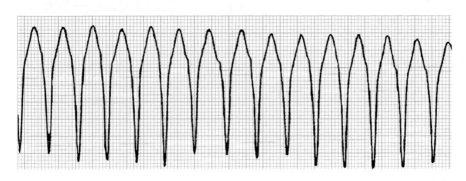

Figure 27.6

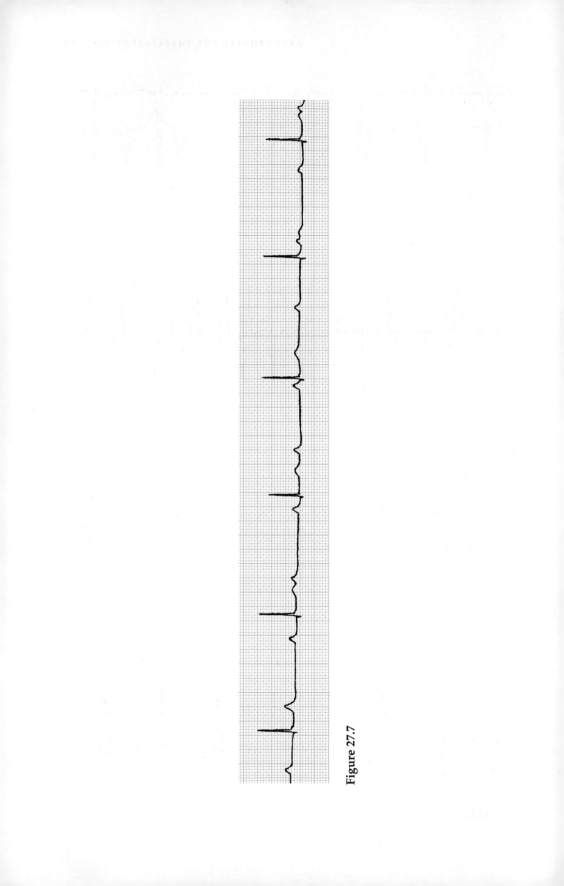

Figure 27.7

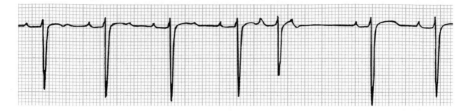

Figure 27.8

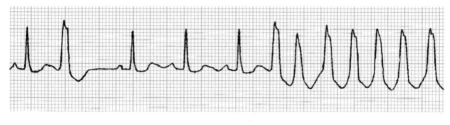

Figure 27.9

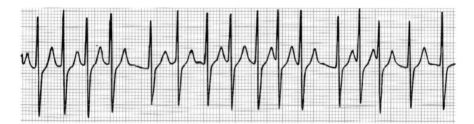

Figure 27.10

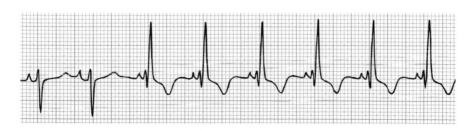

Figure 27.11

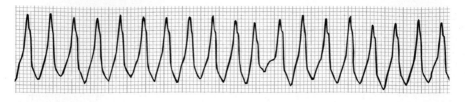

Figure 27.12

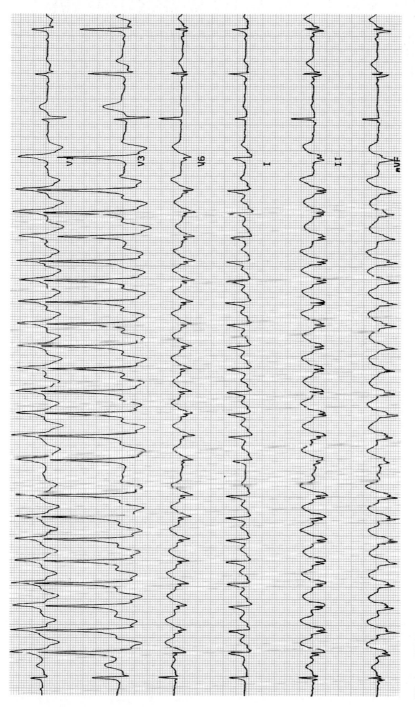

Figure 27.13

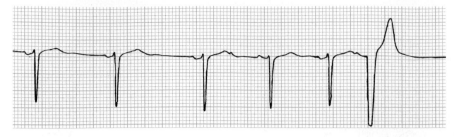

Figure 27.14

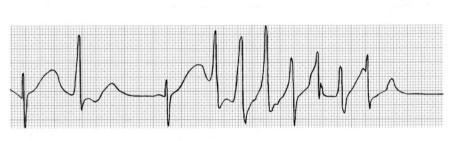

Figure 27.15

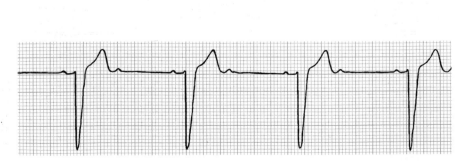

Figure 27.16

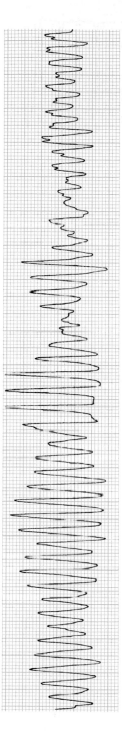

Figure 27.17

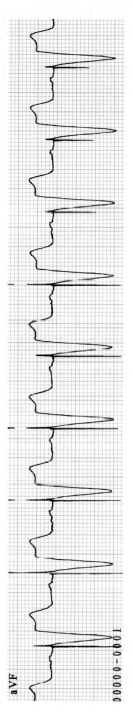

aVF

00000-0001

Figure 27.18

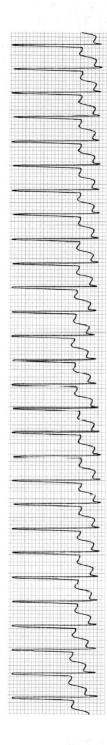

Figure 27.19

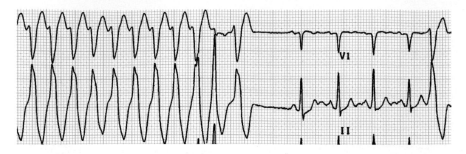

Figure 27.20

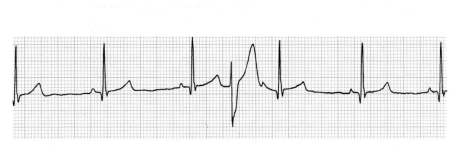

Figure 27.21

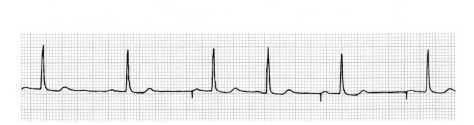

Figure 27.22

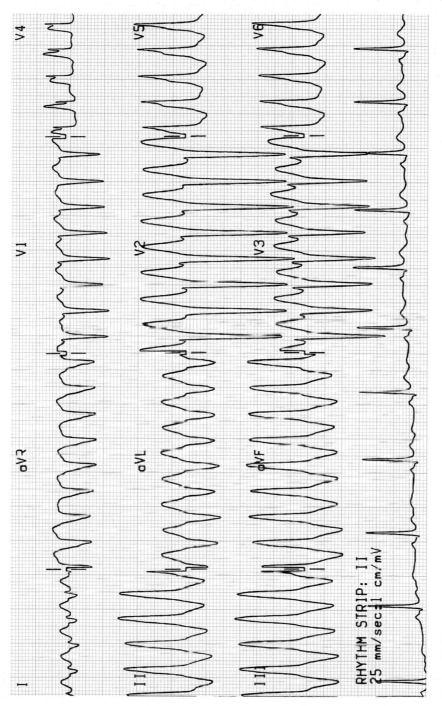

Figure 27.23

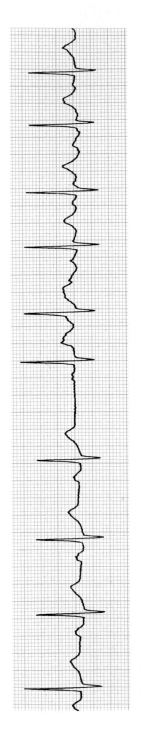

Figure 27.24

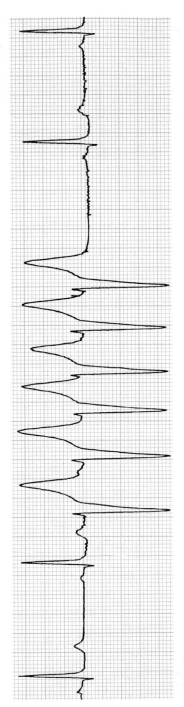

Figure 27.25

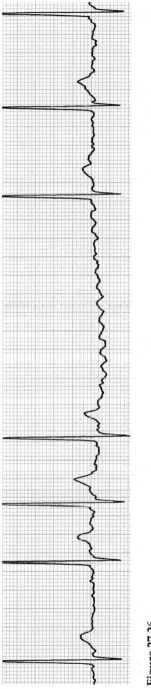

Figure 27.26

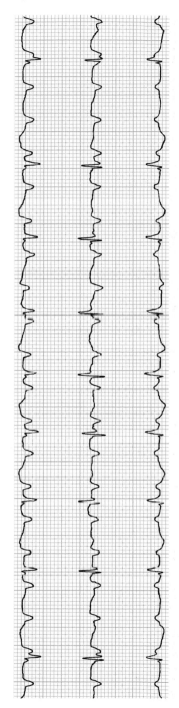

Figure 27.27

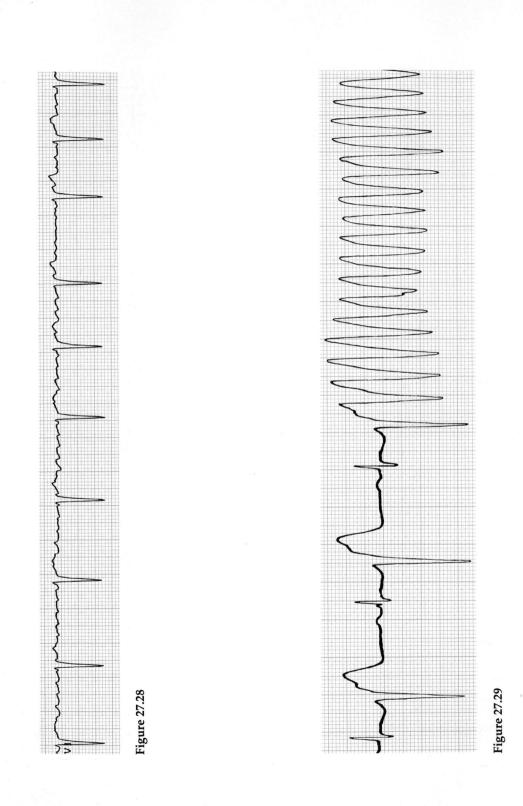

Figure 27.28

Figure 27.29

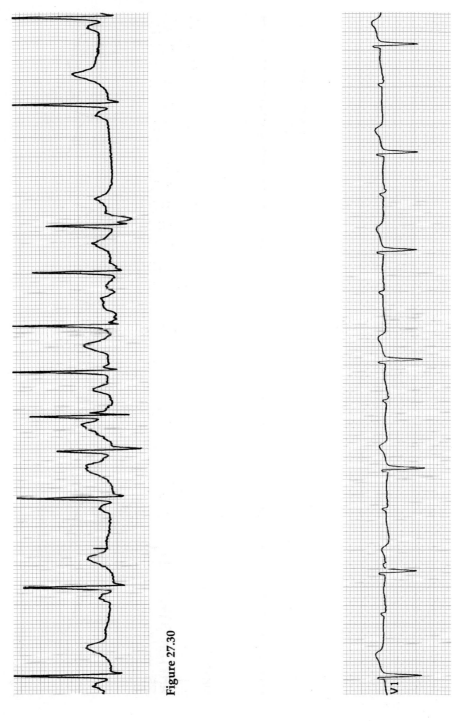

Figure 27.30

Figure 27.31

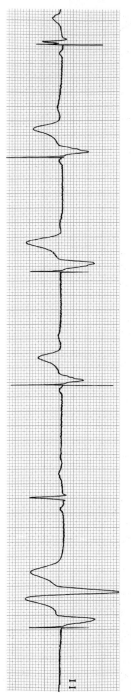

II

Figure 27.32

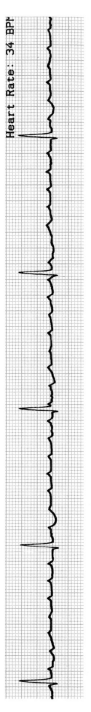

Figure 27.33

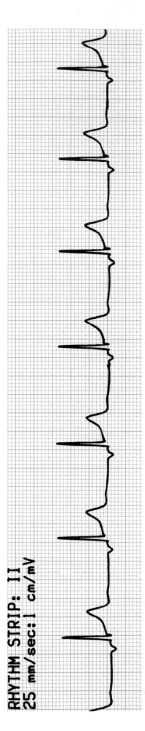

RHYTHM STRIP: II
25 mm/sec:1 cm/mV

Figure 27.34

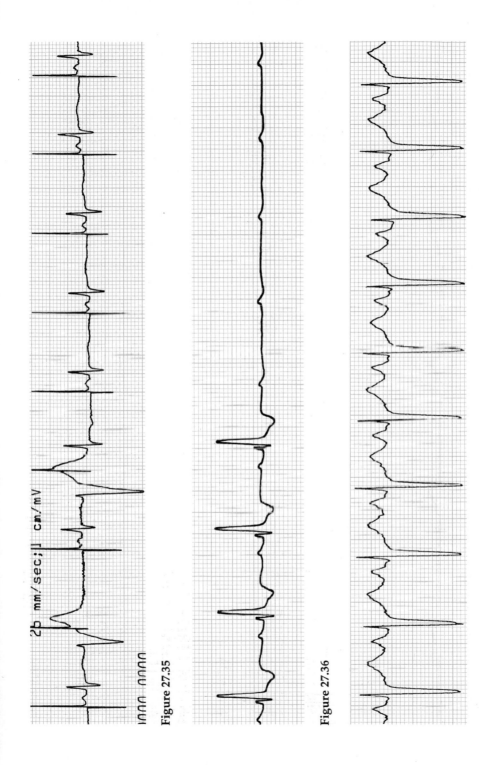

Figure 27.35

Figure 27.36

Figure 27.37

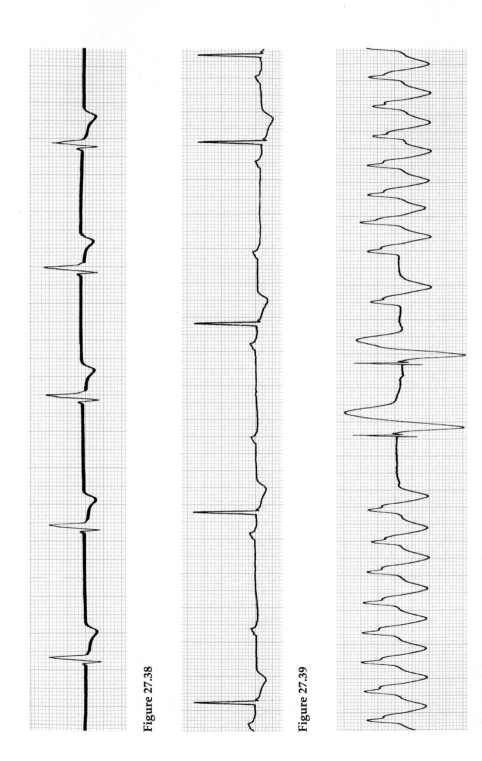

Figure 27.38

Figure 27.39

Figure 27.40

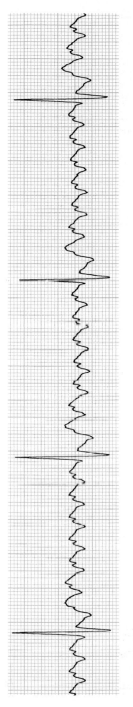

Figure 27.41

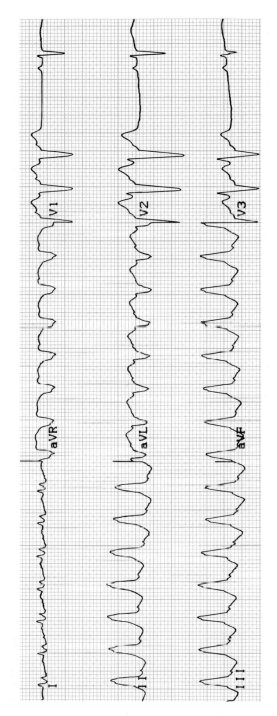

Figure 27.42

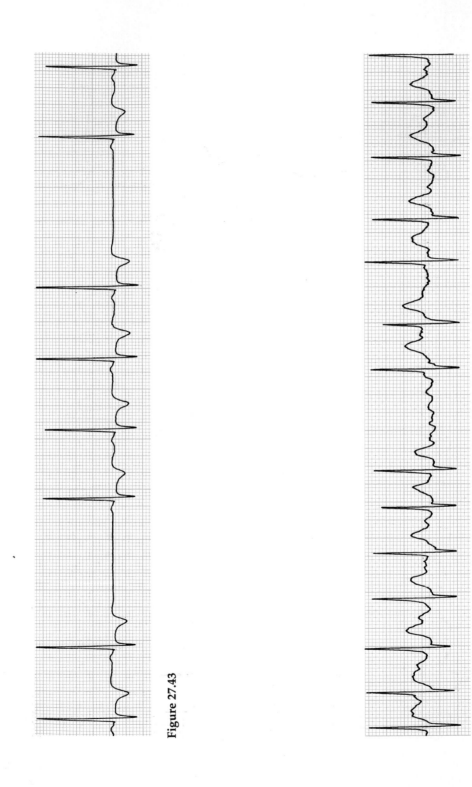

Figure 27.43

Figure 27.44

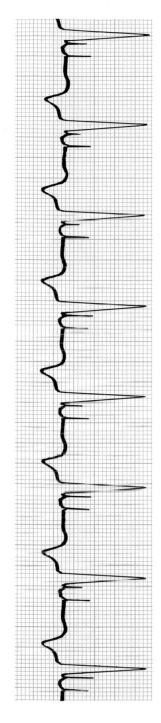

Figure 27.45

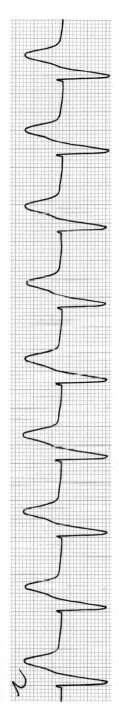

Figure 27.46

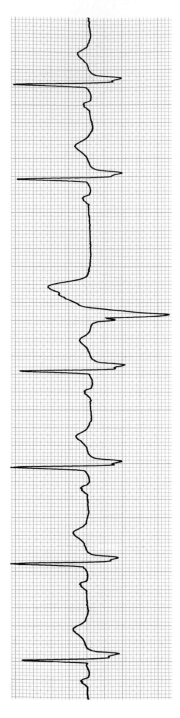

Figure 27.47

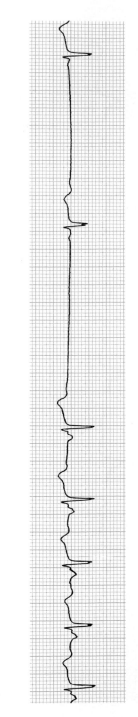

Figure 27.48

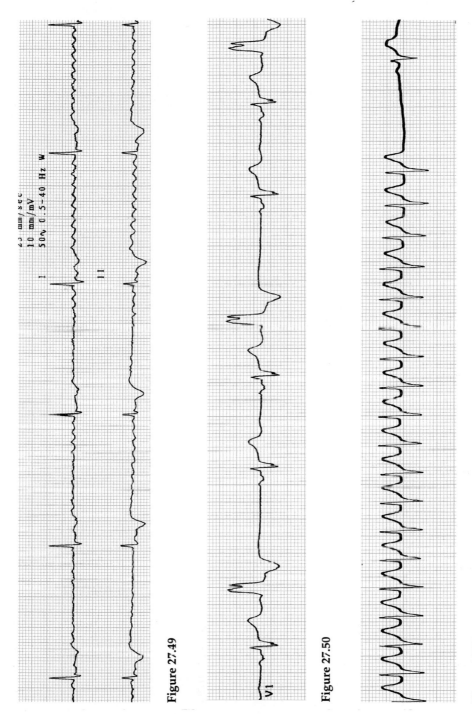

Figure 27.49

Figure 27.50

Figure 27.51

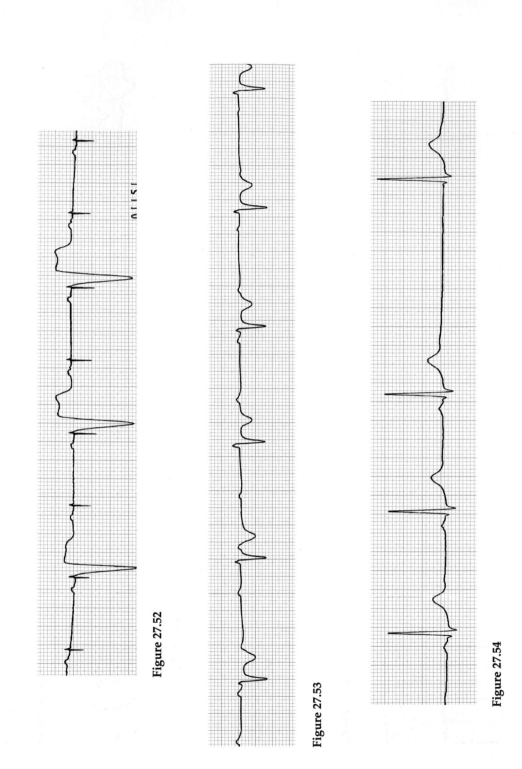

Figure 27.52

Figure 27.53

Figure 27.54

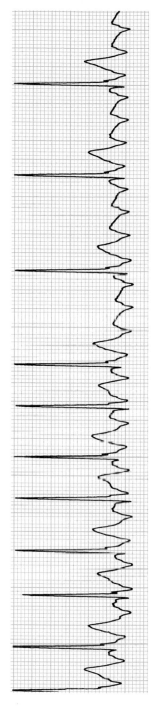

Figure 27.55

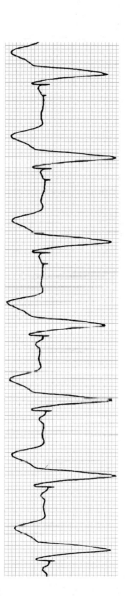

Figure 27.56

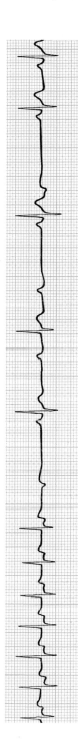

Figure 27.57

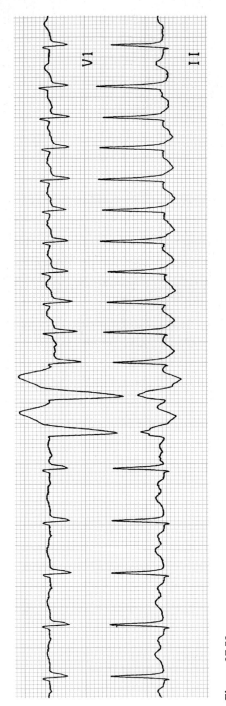

Figure 27.58

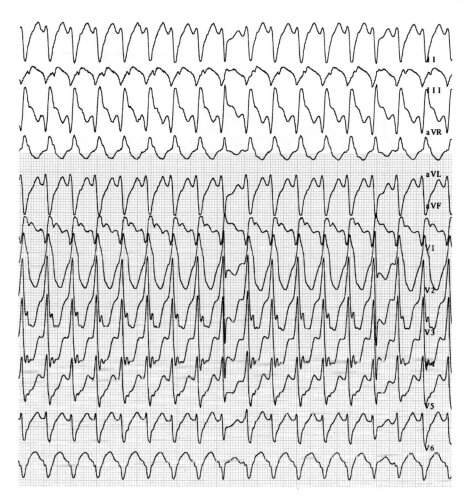

Figure 27.59

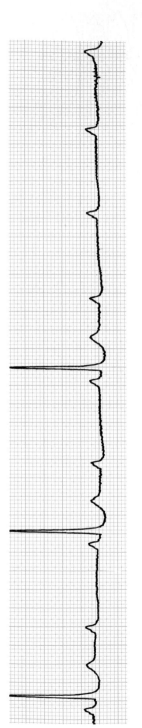

Figure 27.60

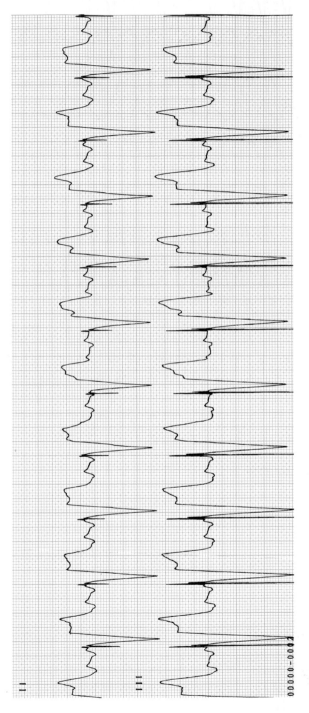

Figure 27.61

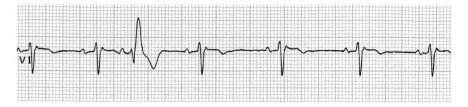

Figure 27.62

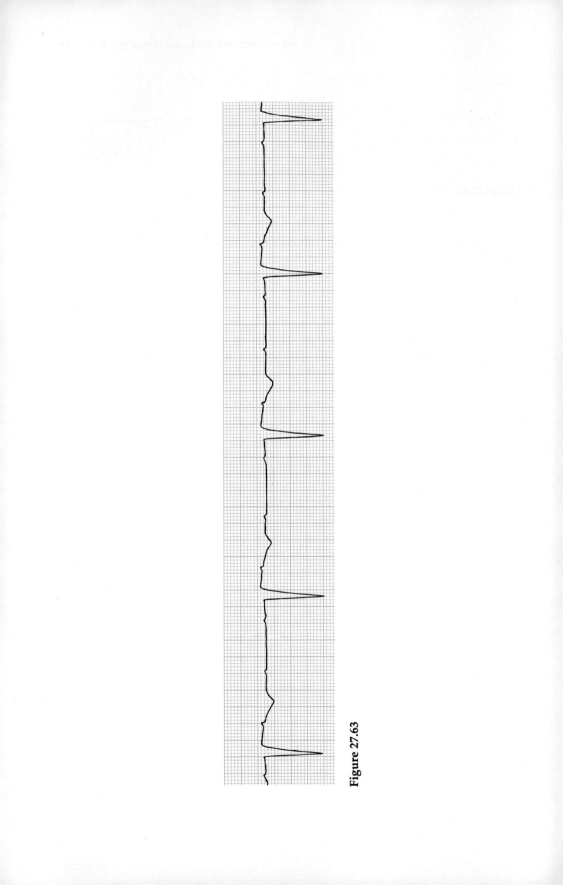

Figure 27.63

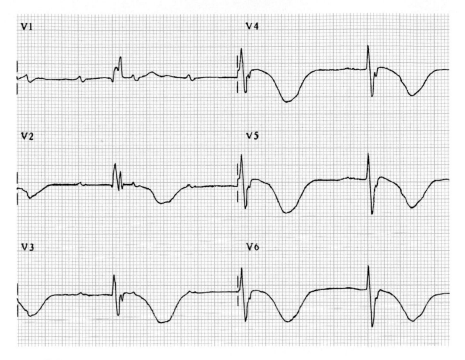

Figure 27.64

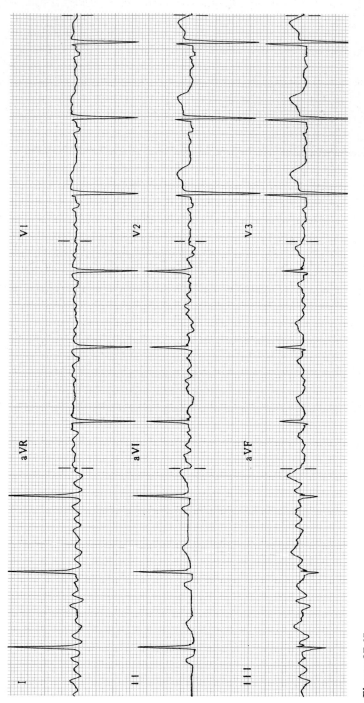

Figure 27.65

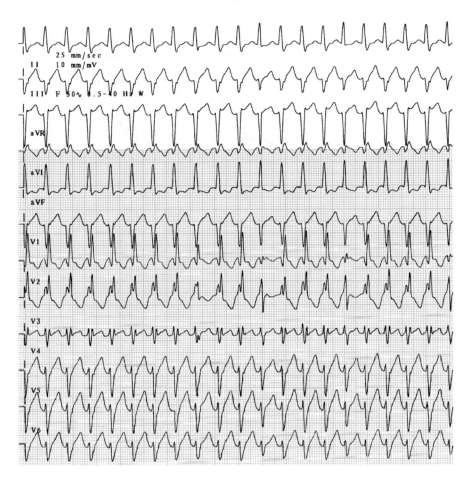

Figure 27.66

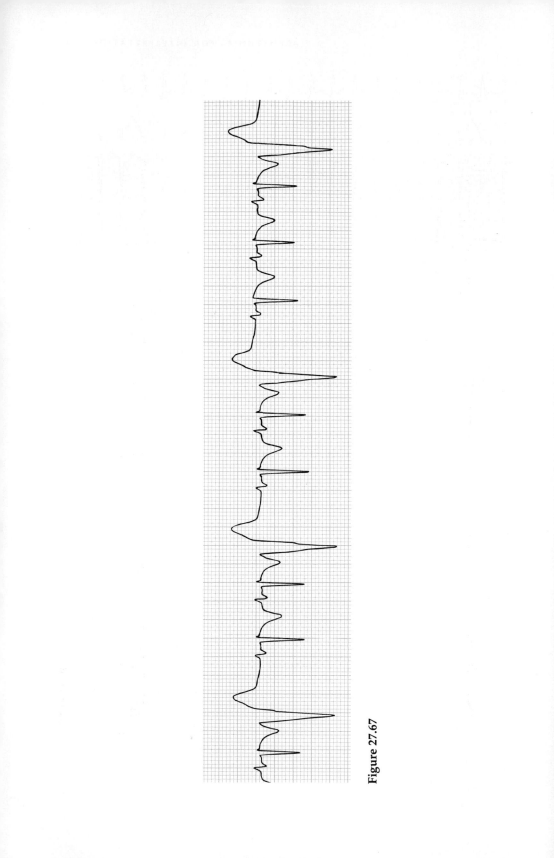

Figure 27.67

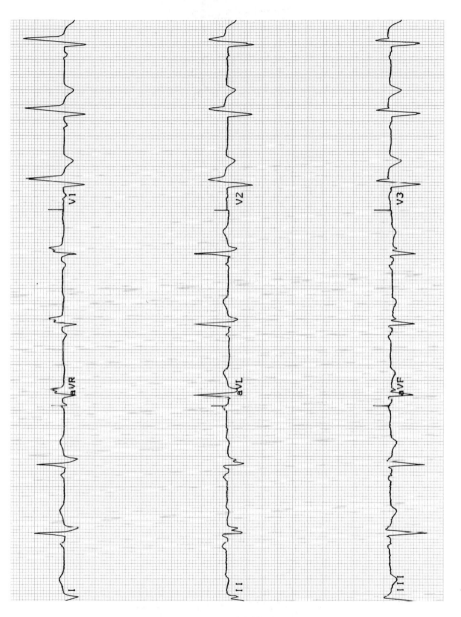

Figure 27.68

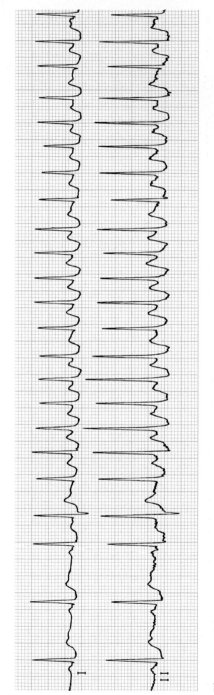

Figure 27.69

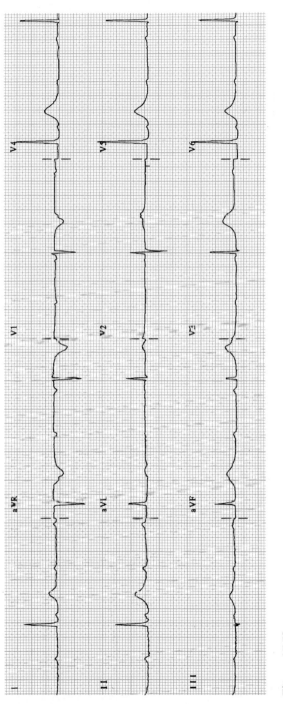

Figure 27.70

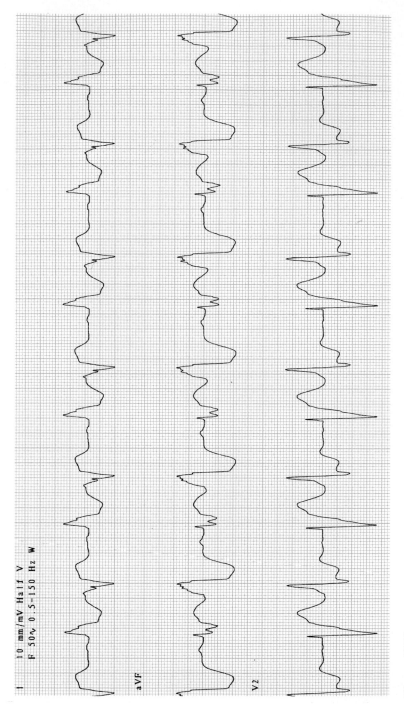

I   10 mm/mV Half V
F 50√ 0.5-150 Hz W

aVF

V2

Figure 27.71

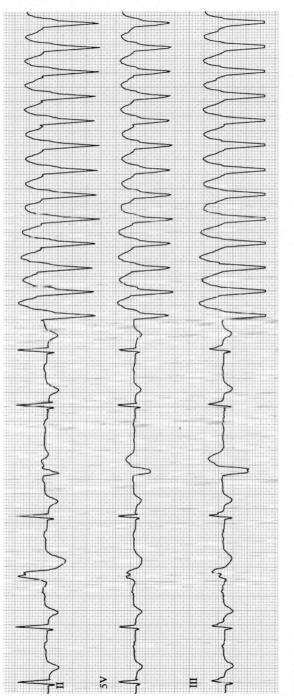

Figure 27.72

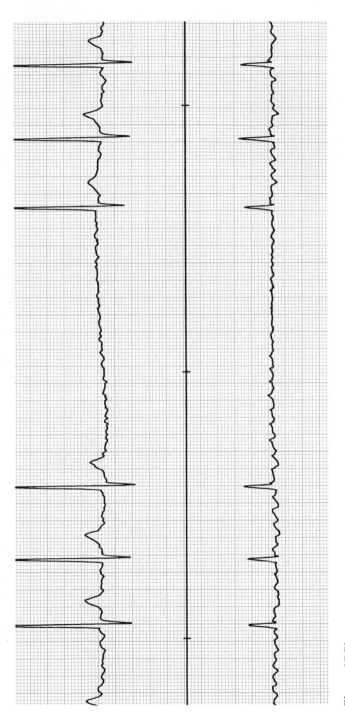

Figure 27.73

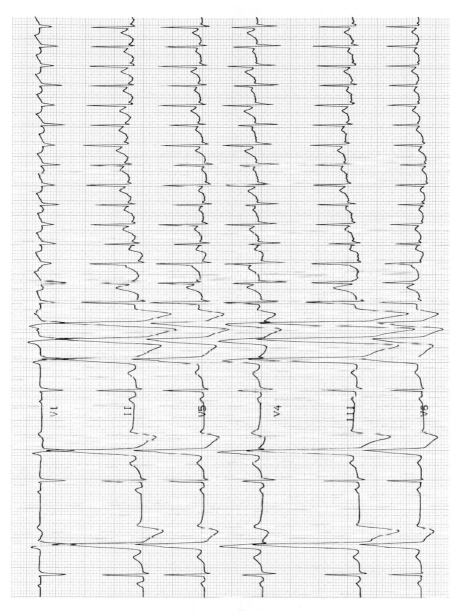

Figure 27.74

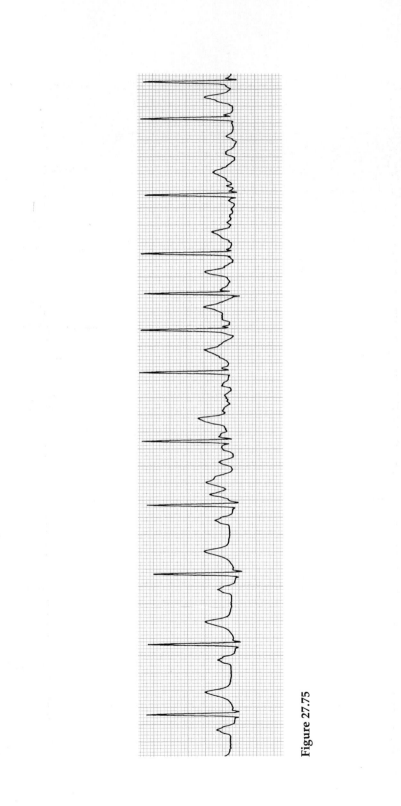

Figure 27.75

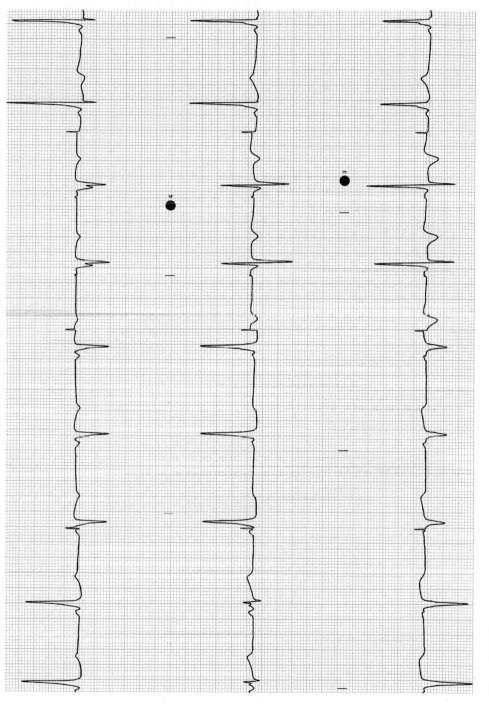

Figure 27.76

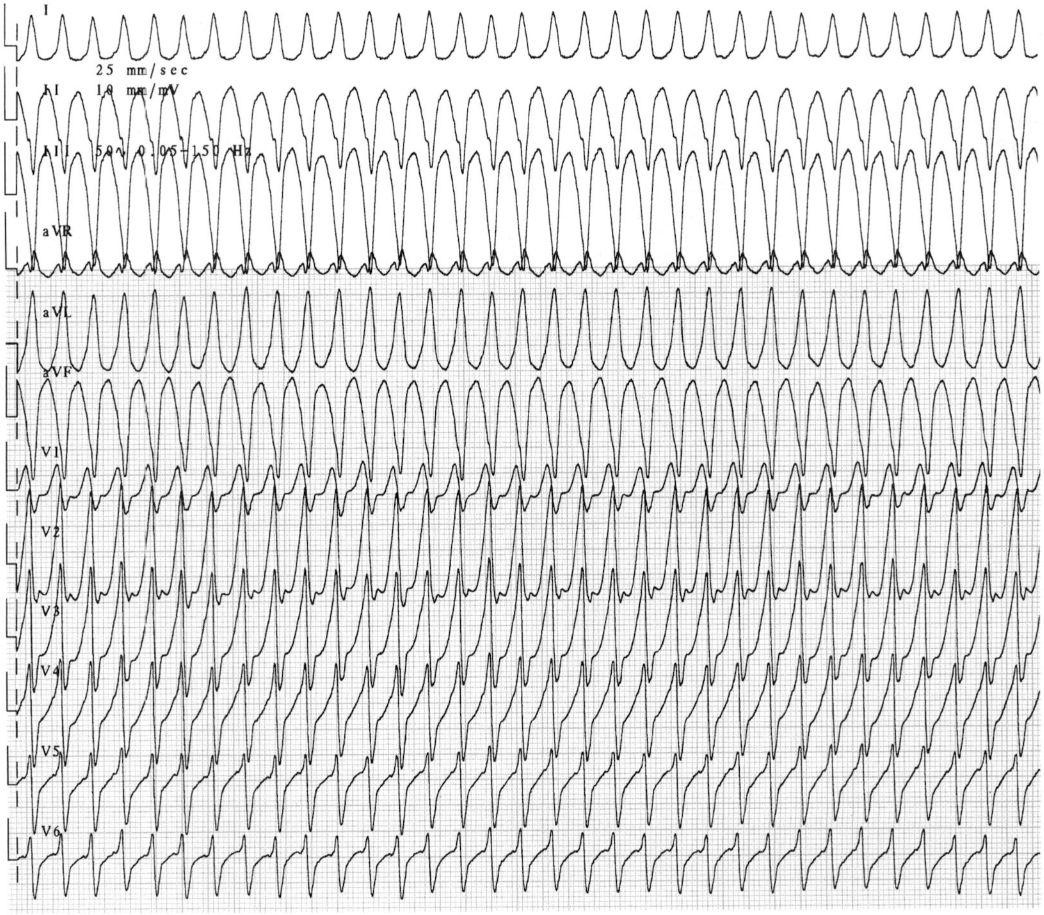

Figure 27.77

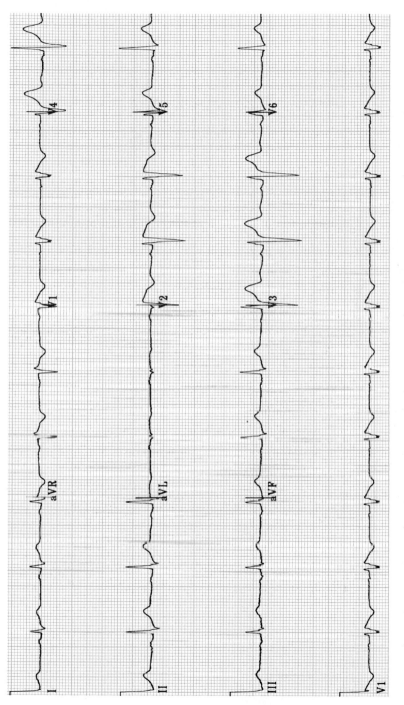

Figure 27.78

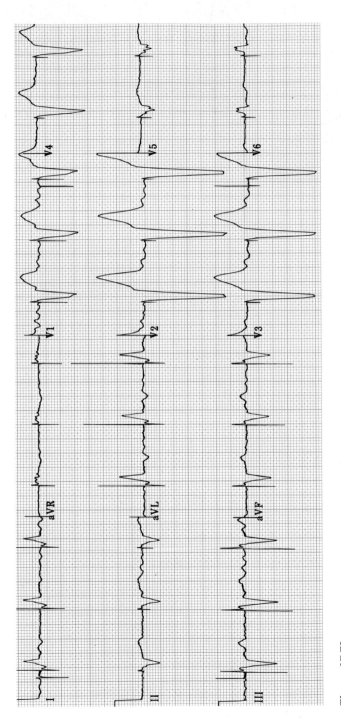

Figure 27.79

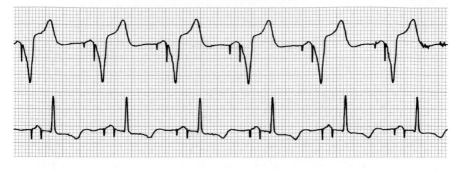

Figure 27.80

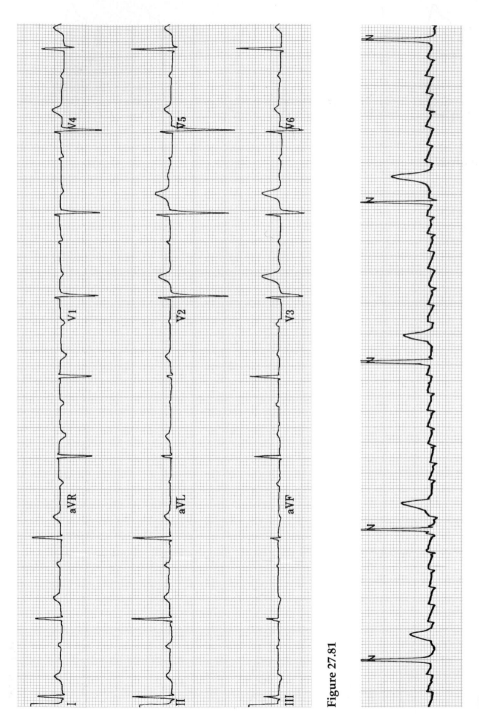

Figure 27.81

Figure 27.82

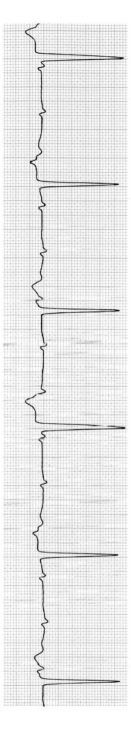

Figure 27.83

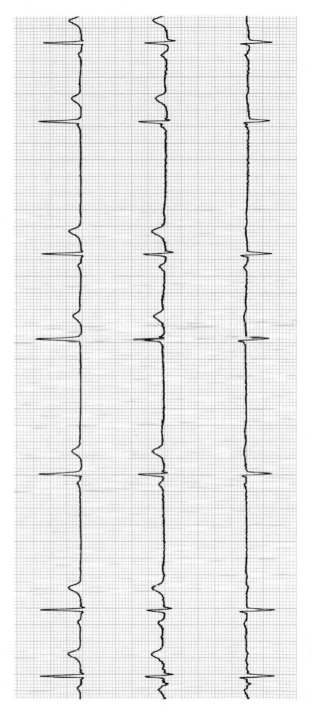

Figure 27.84

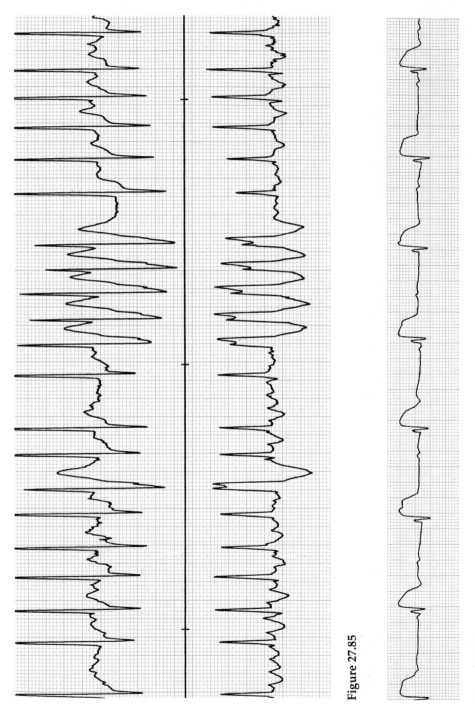

Figure 27.85

Figure 27.86

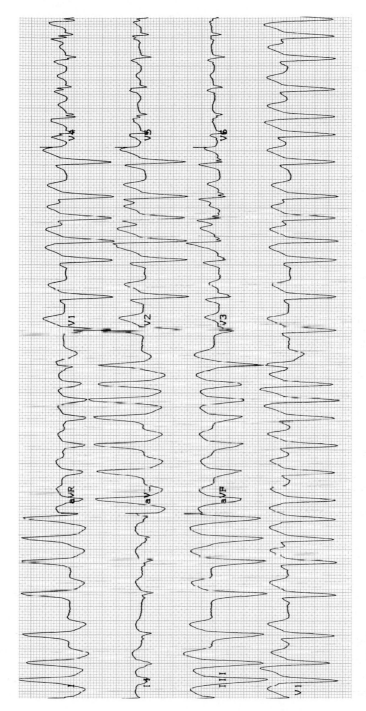

Figure 27.87

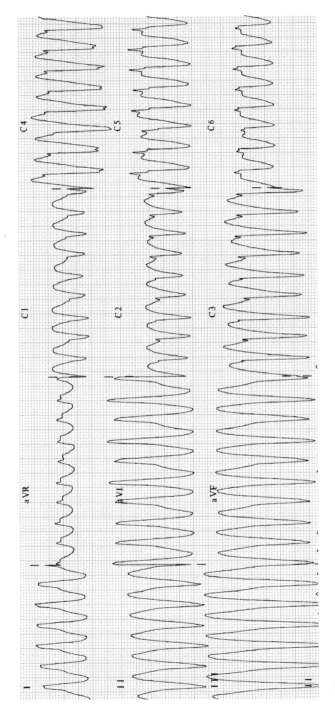

Figure 27.88

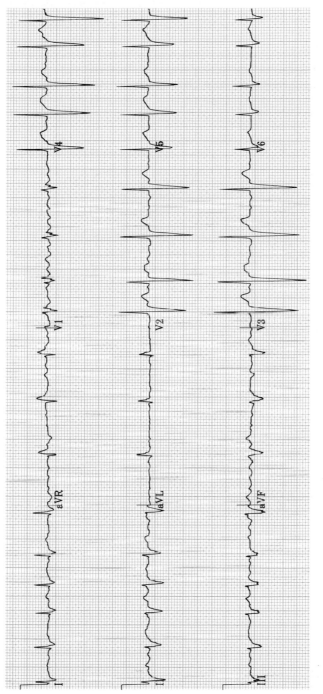

Figure 27.89

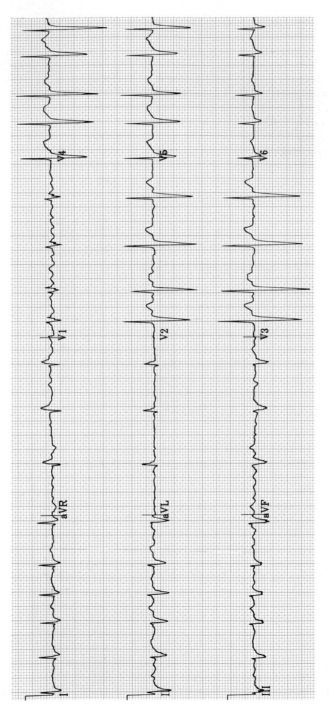

Figure 27.90

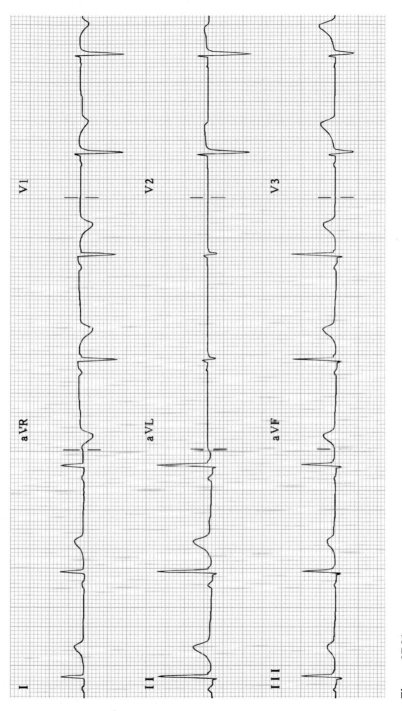

Figure 27.91

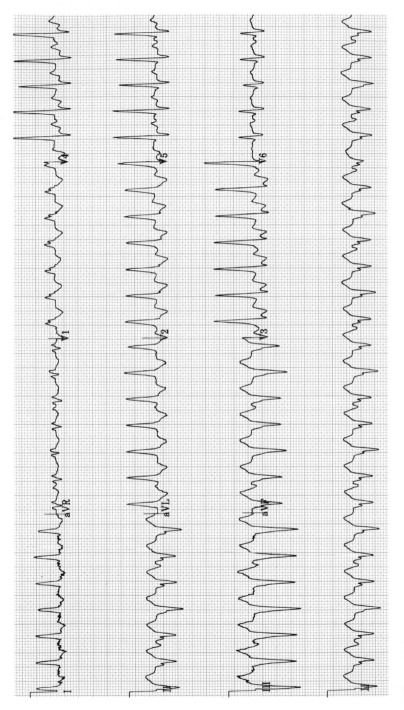

Figure 27.92

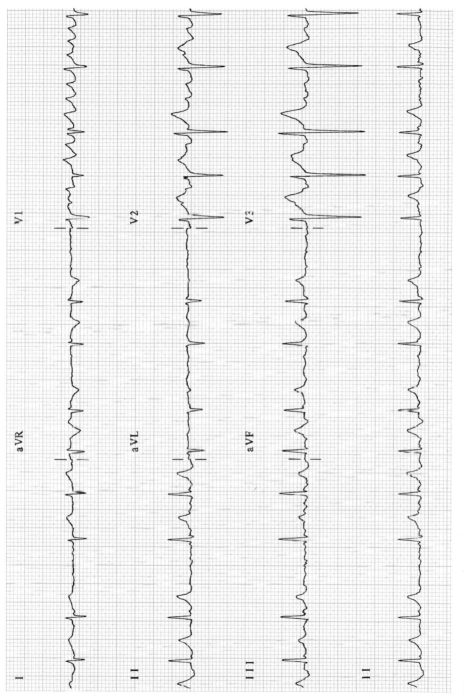

Figure 27.93

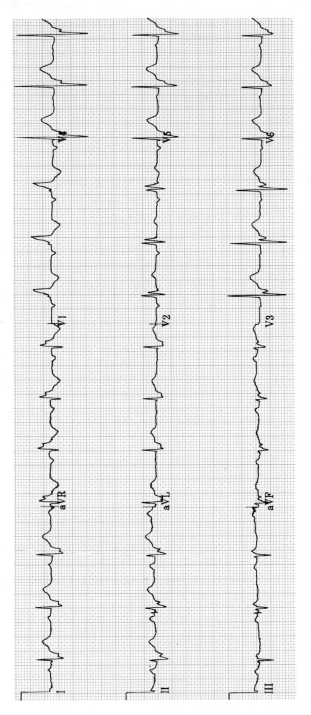

Figure 27.94

INTERPRETATIONS

Figure 27.1 Atrial flutter with 2:1 AV block

Figure 27.2 Sinus rhythm with ventricular trigeminy

Figure 27.3 Ventricular tachycardia. The 16th complex is a fusion beat

Figure 27.4 Ventricular demand pacemaker inhibited by sinus beats. The sixth complex is a fusion beat

Figure 27.5 2:1 AV block with ventricular ectopic beats

Figure 27.6 Ventricular tachycardia

Figure 27.7 Complete AV block with narrow ventricular complexes

Figure 27.8 Atrial ectopic beat superimposed on T wave of fourth ventricular complex. There is a further atrial ectopic beat superimposed on the T wave of the fifth complex which is not conducted to the ventricles

Figure 27.9 The second ventricular ectopic beat initiates ventricular tachycardia

Figure 27.10 Atrial fibrillation with rapid ventricular response

Figure 27.11 After two normally conducted sinus beats there is right bundle branch block (lead V1)

Figure 27.12 Ventricular tachycardia with a fusion beat

Figure 27.13 Paroxysmal atrial fibrillation and Wolff–Parkinson–White syndrome

Figure 27.14 Atrial ectopic beats superimposed on third and fifth ventricular T waves. First ectopic beat is not conducted; the second is conducted to the ventricles with left bundle branch block

Figure 27.15 Sinus bradycardia with long QT interval and short episode of torsade de pointes tachycardia

Figure 27.16 2:1 AV block

Figure 27.17 Ventricular fibrillation

Figure 27.18 Atrial synchronized ventricular pacing

Figure 27.19 AV re-entrant tachycardia

Figure 27.20 Termination of ventricular tachycardia followed by four sinus beats and a ventricular ectopic beat

Figure 27.21 The fourth ventricular complex is an interpolated ventricular ectopic beat

Figure 27.22 Atrial demand pacemaker

Figure 27.23 12-lead ECG showing right ventricular outflow tract tachycardia. Sinus rhythm has returned at time of recording rhythm strip

Figure 27.24 Atrial fibrillation after five sinus beats

Figure 27.25 Short episode of ventricular tachycardia

Figure 27.26 Atrial fibrillation with long pause in ventricular activity

Figure 27.27 Atrial tachycardia with AV block

Figure 27.28 Atrial fibrillation

Figure 27.29 Ventricular tachycardia initiated by third ventricular ectopic beat

Figure 27.30 Paroxysmal atrial fibrillation

Figure 27.31 First degree AV block. PR interval = 0.46 s

Figure 27.32 Ventricular demand pacing at 40 beats/min. Ventricular ectopic after first paced beat. Last complex is a fusion beat

Figure 27.33 Atrial flutter with complete AV block

Figure 27.34 Junctional rhythm

Figure 27.35 Atrial pacing. There are two ventricular ectopic beats which are, of course, not sensed by the pacemaker

Figure 27.36 Ventricular asystole after four sinus beats conducted with right bundle branch block

Figure 27.37 Sinus tachycardia

Figure 27.38 Junctional rhythm

Figure 27.39 Mobitz II AV block

Figure 27.40 Two paced ventricular beats preceded and succeeded by ventricular tachycardia

Figure 27.41 Atrial flutter with high degree AV block

Figure 27.42 Ventricular tachycardia with retrograde atrial activation. Sinus rhythm returns at the end of the ECG

Figure 27.43 Two episodes of second-degree sino-atrial block

Figure 27.44 Atrial fibrillation

Figure 27.45 AV sequential pacing

Figure 27.46 Idioventricular rhythm

Figure 27.47 Single ventricular ectopic beat. First degree AV block

Figure 27.48 Junctional rhythm followed by sinus arrest and then sinus bradycardia

Figure 27.49 Atrial fibrillation and complete AV block

Figure 27.50 Ventricular trigeminy

Figure 27.51 Termination of AV re-entrant tachycardia

Figure 27.52 Ventricular pacing with intermittent failure to capture

Figure 27.53 Complete AV block

Figure 27.54 Sinus arrest followed by junctional escape beat

Figure 27.55 Atrial flutter with varying AV conduction

Figure 27.56 Atrial synchronized and then AV sequential pacing, i.e. DDD pacemaker

Figure 27.57 Complete heart block following termination of supraventricular tachycardia, suggesting that adenosine has been given

Figure 27.58 Onset of AV re-entrant tachycardia following couplet of ventricular ectopic beats

Figure 27.59 Ventricular tachycardia with fusion beats

Figure 27.60 Mobitz II AV block deteriorating to third-degree AV block

Figure 27.61 Atrial flutter; ventricular pacing

Figure 27.62 Incomplete right bundle branch block. The third complex is an atrial ectopic beat, conducted with complete right bundle branch block

Figure 27.63 Mobitz II AV block: there is 3:1 AV conduction

Figure 27.64 Complete AV block, best seen in V1, and marked QT prolongation. (Patient presented with torsade de pointes tachycardia)

Figure 27.65 Normal sinus rhythm. Apparent atrial fibrillation in some of the limb leads due to patient tremor

Figure 27.66 Fusion beats indicate ventricular tachycardia. Relatively narrow QRS complexes together with right bundle branch block and left axis deviation indicate left posterior fascicular origin. 9th, 13th and 17th complexes are capture beats

Figure 27.67 Frequent ventricular ectopic beats

Figure 27.68 Bifascicular block due to anterior myocardial infarction

Figure 27.69 Onset of atrial fibrillation

Figure 27.70 Complete AV block; narrow QRS complexes. QT prolongation = 0.6 s

Figure 27.71 Sinus rhythm, marked QRS prolongation and ventricular bigeminy

Figure 27.72 Mulitfocal ventricular ectopic beats: the third, fifth and eighth complexes. The first is an end-diastolic ectopic beat; the third initiates monomorphic ventricular tachycardia

Figure 27.73 Atrial fibrillation with a very long pause

Figure 27.74 Right ventricular outflow tract bigeminy, then salvo initiates AV re-entrant supraventricular tachycardia

Figure 27.75 Onset of atrial fibrillation after four sinus beats

Figure 27.76 Type B Wolff–Parkinson–White syndrome

Figure 27.77 Monomorphic ventricular tachycardia

Figure 27.78 Brugada syndrome

Figure 27.79 Ventricular pacing; atrial fibrillation

Figure 27.80 Upper trace: AV sequential pacing. Lower trace: failure of ventricular capture

Figure 27.81 First-degree AV block

Figure 27.82 Atrial flutter and complete AV block

Figure 27.83 Complete AV block

Figure 27.84 Sinus arrest followed by junctional escape beats

Figure 27.85 Atrial fibrillation; some broad QRS complexes due to aberrant conduction

Figure 27.86 Lead aVF: complete AV block due to acute inferior infarction

Figure 27.87 Atrial fibrillation. QRS complex appearance strongly suggests Wolff–Parkinson–White syndrome

Figure 27.88 Monomorphic ventricular tachycardia

Figure 27.89 Atrial flutter with 2:1 AV conduction

Figure 27.90 Atrial fibrillation. Left anterior fascicular block and partial right bundle branch block

Figure 27.91 Normal!

Figure 27.92 Ventricular tachycardia with direct evidence of independent P waves

Figure 27.93 Atrial fibrillation

Figure 27.94 Left anterior hemiblock and right bundle branch block

Note: 'vs ' indicates the differentiation of two or more conditions. Abbreviations: MI, myocardial infarction